SEARCHING FOR HEALING

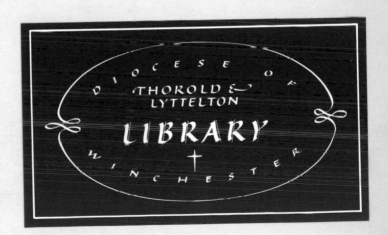

Searching For Healing

Making sense of the many paths to wholeness

STEPHEN PARSONS

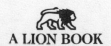

A LION BOOK

Published by
Lion Publishing plc
Sandy Lane West, Oxford, England
ISBN 0 7459 3127 8
Albatross Books Pty Ltd
PO Box 320, Sutherland, NSW 2232, Australia
ISBN 0 7324 1308 7

First edition 1995

10 9 8 7 6 5 4 3 2 1 0

A catalogue record for this book is available
from the British Library

Printed and bound in Great Britain
by Cox & Wyman Ltd, Reading

Contents

ACKNOWLEDGMENTS

This book is the result of discussions and reading over the past ten years. I am particularly grateful to my association with the Churches' Council for Health and Healing for the stimulus it has provided to me to think about healing issues over the last four years. I am also thankful to Maurice Lyon of Lion Publishing for providing me with the chance to set my ideas down on paper. I am aware that many conversations that I have had with individuals have fed into these ideas and I gratefully acknowledge them even though many of the occasions are now forgotten. Three people provided help with the manuscript and made valuable suggestions for improvements of style and accuracy: Professor John Webb, Dorothy Dickinson and Yvonne Wells. The creation of any book involves absences from other responsibilities and I am grateful to my parish of St Lawrence Lechlade for not missing me too much for the greater part of January 1995 while I was completing the text. Above all I acknowledge the support of my family for their understanding during my hours in my study in front of the word processor. It is to them, Frances, Anna and Clare, that this book is dedicated.

Introduction

There are few subjects which exercise such a universal fascination as that of health and healing. Listen to a conversation between two elderly people and likely as not it will be about their latest diagnosed complaint. From the discussion about symptoms the conversation may well turn to methods of cure. Depending on the background of the person speaking, a number of remedies will be aired ranging from the conventional to the superstitious or strange. One does not have to listen to many such conversations today to realize that few people are unaffected by one or other of the 'alternative' cultures of healing that abound in our society.

Medical practitioners will be puzzled or irritated by some of the ideas from these other cultures that patients cling on to. Whatever else is true, medical science is no longer perceived by many people to be the only resource for healing. Although it holds the high ground in terms of prestige and power, it has to coexist with many other lesser cultures of healing. The word 'culture' presupposes a distinctive set of ideas and assumptions behind it. Much to the mystification of the official purveyors of health to our society, those in the medical profession, these ideas and assumptions often have little in common with the norms and values that they have been taught to hold.

This book is a study of the cultures of healing in our society. It makes no attempt to be comprehensive or complete. But it does seek to offer some understanding of the background ideas that undergird each of these cultures. Some come out of religious beliefs, others find their meaning in various esoteric philosophical systems. In presenting all these sets of beliefs and ideas alongside one another, I hope to foster a better mutual comprehension between the cultures both for patients and therapists.

It is difficult to set out on a journey to visit strange places without a map. The map that is provided for the reader, because it is written by a Christian author, gives Christian methods of healing an honoured place amid all the other cultures and styles examined, but in no way suggests that other methods and styles of healing should be written off because they are outside the boundaries of Christian belief. Neither are conclusions drawn as to the effectiveness of different therapies in promoting healing. This book presents a map of new roads that sadly did not appear on many older maps drawn by Christians of the same territory. It is along these new roads that fresh understanding and tolerance may travel, so that the old ways of confrontation and conflict can be lessened.

A note to those who are ill

There may be some readers who start this book in the hope that it may contain some solutions or suggestions for the healing of their own particular problem. However, the intention of the author has not been to set out ideas for solving detailed problems of health. There has been a broader aim: to set out a variety of ways of thinking about healing by exploring the range of models within our contemporary society which seek to provide health and healing. Readers may well after finishing this book be encouraged to look wider beyond a single culture for solutions to their problems. Here a word of warning should be offered. Just as many people who occupy the medical perspective on health think only of medical solutions to problems of sickness, so there are many in the alternative healing cultures who claim to offer the only answer. Be very suspicious of anyone who claims to have the whole truth in matters of healing. It is very unlikely to be true. Responsible people involved in healing, whether Christian, medical or alternative, know that the mystery of the human body and spirit is far greater than any single body of truth or culture can contain. I wish you well in your search for health. It will require determination, discernment and time, and the search for healing may not ultimately restore full health, but it may provide you with new resources and a discovery of new aspects of your personality that you never knew before. Christians have always recognized that illness and weakness can be used for a greater good if we allow them to do so. As Paul discovered when battling with his 'thorn in the flesh', God's power is 'made perfect in weakness'.

CHAPTER 1

Healing with Medicine

In trying to understand any healing system or technique in our society we have to begin with one simple reality. Nature has put into all living things, plants, animals and human beings, certain complex mechanisms which allow damage to be repaired, infection to be defeated and the whole equilibrium of the organism to be restored. In short we all possess a capacity to heal ourselves by allowing nature to do its work of restoration and repair. Those who study these internal mechanisms of healing will have cause to wonder at the sheer beauty and perfection of these processes. Another word that can be used is 'wisdom'. The body has genetically imprinted within it a knowledge of how to overcome the effects of disease and injury in many different ways Unless our bodily functioning is weakened by malnutrition or chronic disease, these mechanisms will work every time without any effort or thought on our part.

The healing arts today all begin with this capacity of the body to fight illness and, in the majority of cases, produce healing for itself. In different ways the healing arts encourage and assist this process and in some cases make up what the body itself lacks to effect healing. Although co-operation with the body in its attempts to find its own healing would appear to be common sense, medical practice has not always followed this principle. Until the middle of the nineteenth century a doctor trained in Western medicine would be far more likely to assault the body with purgatives, bleeding or cupping as a way of stimulating it to fight disease. The understanding of the body's own methods of fighting disease has only relatively recently become part of medical knowledge and treatment.

The success of medicine in the last forty years, in particular, has been built on the ability of the medical profession to understand countless processes within the body for preserving and promoting health and to discover how to enhance and assist these processes. Medicine, in short, is the science of understanding the processes of healing in the body and providing the necessary stimuli, surgical or chemical, to make those healings more likely to take place. The success of the discipline in promoting health has meant that it has taken a position of pre-eminence in the Western world over all other methods of healing. This success and the power that follows it, however, have left conventional medicine neither unchallenged nor without rivals. While those who do challenge it are usually among the first to recognize its many achievements, they perceive weakness at a deeper level, the level of basic assumptions about the human body and mind.

The culture of medicine

Medical science and research over the past two hundred years share, in common with the whole of modern science, a set of particular philosophical premises which were developed in the seventeenth and eighteenth centuries. In brief there is an assumption in both science and the technology that emerges from it that the nature of an object is ultimately understood by 'reductionist' or 'mechanistic' means, breaking it down to its constituent parts. Medicine shares this basic philosophical premise. Progress in understanding the human body has been achieved by the study of the large number of independent systems within it, each of which can be treated independently.

Obviously, in practice, interrelationships between the different parts of the body are recognized but it is worth commenting on how many of the specialties within medicine are for particular areas of the body. Such specialization is inevitable and indeed desirable, because it is difficult for any one person to master the enormous amount of knowledge required to understand fully the workings of even a small section of the body. A narrow concentration on particular parts of the body in diagnosis and treatment is a distinctive feature of medicine but emerges in part from the reductionist philosophy that undergirds the whole enterprise.

Within medical practice the most important implication of dividing a patient into separate parts is when the body and mind are treated as distinct and independent. The idea that the body should be set free from the shackles of the mind so that it can be examined quite separately is, in particular, the result of the philosophical speculations of a seventeenth-century Frenchman, René Descartes. He was concerned with the issue of examining the world around him without having to take into account the accretions of the traditional beliefs that had grown up over the centuries. In short, he wanted to be able to examine the world around him objectively without the subjectivity of beliefs and feelings intruding on what was found. He proposed that the conscious mind be sundered from everything else so that only facts which had been objectively measured would be counted as real knowledge.

This discipline of objective measurement not only became the method of working for scientists like Isaac Newton and all who have followed him but it also changed the way that ordinary men and women within Western culture saw the world. Objectivity, experiment and free enquiry were to be the marks of proper scientific enquiry. The method was rapidly extended to include all other areas of knowledge. When such a way of 'seeing' was applied to the human being,, it naturally concentrated on the measurable aspects of the individual, the physical body. Thus medical science came to regard the problems of illness in mechanistic terms and its treatment as the repair of a broken machine.

The centuries following Descartes, while further encouraging doctors to study the body's mechanical aspects (something they had been forbidden to do in the Middle Ages for religious reasons), did not at first produce a great deal to help people to recover from their illnesses. The discovery of bacterial organisms in the nineteenth century was a boost to the scientific medical model and further confirmation that both the body and its disease processes were explicable in terms of a machine. Along with these new theories came the possibility of safe surgery with higher standards of hygiene. The systematic development of vaccines also proved effective in preventing some of the much feared infectious diseases of the day such as tetanus and diphtheria. New levels of hygiene and nutrition in society as a whole also made a fairly dramatic contribution to the slow defeat of other endemic diseases such as tuberculosis.

Few effective drug treatments existed at the turn of the century once such diseases had taken hold. One nineteenth century physician, Oliver Wendel Holmes, commented that if the entire contents of the current pharmacopoeia were tipped into the sea it would be all the better for mankind and all the worse for the fishes—a fair reflection of the poor state of treatment by drugs until the last fifty or sixty years. This relatively poor showing by conventional medicine in the face of much untreatable illness meant that, in North America at any rate, a long battle with other forms of healing was fought right up into the present century. As we shall see in a later chapter, scientific or clinical medicine in the last century was hard-pressed to maintain its supremacy against other forms of healing which today we would class as 'alternative'.

The great breakthrough for medical science, and a further triumphant confirmation of its mechanistic theories, came in the 1930s and 1940s with the discovery of effective antibiotics such as sulphanilamide and penicillin. At last, doctors could amazingly treat diseases for which no treatment had before been possible.

Pneumonia, diphtheria, childbirth sepsis and tuberculosis all virtually disappeared in the developed world. Alongside these triumphs, surgical techniques made ever-increasing advances with all kinds of new procedures, the most dramatic of which today are the transplants of many organs of the body. On the wave of these successes came the hope that, in time, every illness would either succumb to a 'magic bullet' in the form of an appropriate pill or could be corrected through a surgical technique. It is a hope that still sustains many people in our society, a faith that whatever may happen to them a doctor somewhere will be able to bring them back to full health. A hope of this kind must be endemic in a society where, against all the evidence, so many people continue to believe that they have nothing to fear from smoking.

The model of the human body in conventional medicine, however, is not one that is unchallenged today. Thirty years ago, few questioned the materialist bias of medicine and its tendency to look at the body as a machine without reference to either environmental or mental processes. What has changed in the last twenty or thirty years both within and beyond the profession is the realization that the old ways of thinking about the human body are based not on some infallible and unchangeable wisdom but on premises that are capable of being questioned. Traditional medical thinking is giving way to a new insight, now widely shared in our society, that each individual person is a complex unity of body, mind and spirit. Illness is not experienced just as a set of symptoms; it has effects at every level of our being.

Christians have long spoken of human beings as a unity of soul and body, and it seems that many people in our society are now prepared to affirm that health as well as healing have dimensions which go way beyond the level of mere mechanical functioning. Many people now demand care from their doctors which affirms the wholeness of their being, rather than treatments which see them as broken-down machines in need of correction or repair.

The rise of 'alternative' or complementary medicine is as much about seeking for 'soul' in the healing process as about dissatisfaction with the mechanical methods of traditional medical treatment. Medicine itself, though rooted in a philosophy that treats the human being as a complex machine, is moving beyond those roots to recognize a new philosophy that does greater justice to the meaning of human life as a whole.

Healing and the techniques of medicine

The traditional way of regarding the human body as a machine is a model that works in many situations and in many cases works brilliantly. A body with broken bones after an accident needs the patient skill of a surgeon. A cancerous growth blocking digestion or breathing needs instant removal. A fever that is caused by a virulent bacterial infection responds well to the administration of antibiotics. In each of these cases, the body is operating like a machine and mechanical intervention is right and appropriate. Lives are saved and full bodily function is restored. Healing of the affected part is established.

Earlier in the chapter we had a brief glimpse of the body's own capacity for self-healing. At this point we need to look briefly at the ways in which medicine enhances these mechanisms, making healing more likely and more permanent.

A wound will be cleaned, covered and stitched, if necessary, to allow healing to take place speedily and without complication. When an infection is severe, chemical antidotes specific to the bacteria can be administered, speeding up the process of healing and in some cases saving the patient's life. The invading bacteria, to use the analogy of war, are not always defeated by the body's defence systems, especially when the host is weakened by long illness or malnutrition. Whereas a well-nourished child will not often find an attack of measles fatal, the same illness can kill a malnourished child. The antibiotics of today are sometimes life-savers, although they may be used too often for trivial illnesses where the bodily mechanisms are quite adequate for self-healing. Other drugs will check disease processes by working directly on the chemistry of the body, neutralizing the growth of ulcers or inhibiting cancers, for example, or making good a deficiency as insulin does in diabetes.

Beyond the use of drugs, the second broad area of medical activity is the domain of surgery. It is perhaps here that the mechanical model is most obviously relevant. Obstructions in various parts of the body may become apparent and need to be cleared; growths occur and have to be removed; parts of the body wear out and may be replaced. Of all the surgical procedures on offer today, perhaps the most life-changing is the replacement of a hip or knee for the elderly person who suffers from osteoarthritis. Eye surgery, likewise, is miraculous for many people. The medical profession can rightly take enormous pride in the achievements of many surgical operations and the contribution they make to restoring health.

A third important area of medical effort lies in the management of chronic (long-term) illness. Here the emphasis is less on healing but more on the management of symptoms and making life more bearable. Much if not most of a GP's time will be spent in helping individuals, especially the elderly, to learn to live with a host of incurable chronic conditions. Little may be on offer by way of actual therapy which will lead to healing. Instead, pain killers, drugs which reduce symptoms and sympathetic words are handed out so that the patient may adapt to various levels of pain and disability. Medical graduates, trained in hospitals where there were frequent possibilities of active intervention and promotion of the body's own healing systems, are sometimes somewhat disillusioned when they discover how little they can do to cure many of the people who come to the GP's surgery.

The high profile of high-tech medicine is sometimes of little relevance to a wide range of chronic illnesses that exist in our society. But the management of pain is itself a highly valued and important skill, particularly among the dying. One doctor said to me recently that the part of his work that he found the most worthwhile was the care of the dying. His patients were no longer looking to him for cure but for care, and in caring he had a lot to offer—in human love and adequate drugs for the control of pain. Behind this comment may also have been a certain frustration at not being able to meet the expectations of other chronically ill patients who believed that he might be holding back on some new treatment that they deserved.

The limitations of medicine

In this brief review of the culture and practice of medical science we have touched on the fact that our society has come to expect a great deal from doctors which they cannot always deliver. Chronic illnesses like emphysema, Parkinson's disease, asthma, arthritis and high blood pressure cannot yet be cured; rather, they can at best be alleviated and managed. But the popular belief that medicine is about effective therapy leading to *cure* lingers on in many parts of our society. In the face of the strong expectations of their patients, some doctors are tempted to go on treating patients, to show that they are in control of the situation, long after realistic options for real improvement in the condition have been exhausted.

A further myth exists in the minds of the general public about the responsibility of medical doctors for the removal of the causes of illness in our society. Thanks to their training and the philosophy underlying it, doctors have traditionally concentrated on the symptoms and treatment of illness once it has begun, and have only recently begun to get involved in the environmental and social causes of illness. Issues of lifestyle, diet and pollution have only fairly recently become so critical in our society, and many people have retained the illusion that these things are unimportant or, if important, can be corrected by medicines if sickness ensues.

The underlying philosophy of medicine, which has tended to concentrate on looking at the parts of a body rather than looking at the whole person within their environment, can take some responsibility for this. When public bodies, backed up by the medical profession, publish exhortations about diet or the evils of smoking in an attempt to correct this area of neglect in health care, many people do not take them seriously. One reason for this may be that individuals have become so used to accepting the old-fashioned, disease-centred perspective on health that they cannot embrace the quite different approach being put forward by the health promotion bodies.

A second consequence of the philosophy undergirding medical practice, which we looked at in the first section of this chapter, is the traditional role allotted to the patient in the healing relationship. Doctors in the past have particularly preferred that their patients be as passive and accepting as possible. The 'good' patient is the co-operative patient, the one who submits most closely to the model of being a machine on whom others can work their skills, either through drugs or surgery. The word 'patient' itself is a word that comes from the same root as the word 'passive'. We shall see in further chapters that passivity is regarded by other healing cultures as working against healing. What is required is the active and total co-operation of the person who comes seeking healing. A human being in totality also incorporates a spiritual being, and we shall be seeing how the spirit may also be engaged and activated in the search for healing.

The belief that conventional medicine alone will have sufficient resources one day to conquer all ill health is one that burdens the day-to-day work of many doctors. Individuals have been encouraged in this idea by the rapid advances of medical science and the sheer size of the resources which our modern society invests in health care. Failure to deliver good health for all is so often seen as a denial of adequate funds to carry out research in the particular health issues of the day. But if the profession is burdened by unrealistic expectations of what can be delivered in the way of health for all, then to some extent it shares responsibility for the propagation of this belief.

The issue would seem in part to be one of institutional power. When the medical profession was being re-organized in the last century in this country and in the United States, it took great care to exclude what were perceived to be dubious practitioners and 'quack' methods from the profession. But in the process of defining itself as a profession, it took a monopolistic attitude to health care. Both governments and the general public got used to the idea that health was an area which could be completely entrusted to professional doctors and that they need look no further for advice and understanding. The idea that we are all to some extent responsible for our health was not part of the original contract between the medical establishment and its public. The ordinary person, having handed over control in health matters to the professionals, now finds it hard to take back even some of this power and responsibility.

The power exercised by the medical establishment (though not necessarily by individual doctors) is an ethical concern every bit as important as the ethical issues of genetic engineering. Patients may sometimes feel totally intimidated in their relationships with doctors, particularly those at a senior level. The consultation with a GP can all too easily be terminated by the powerful one in the relationship standing up and walking to the door. Sometimes important decisions are made on behalf of a patient without the latter's insight and understanding about his or her condition ever having been really heard. Clearly, power in the doctor–patient relationship is weighted on the side of the doctor, though this is not to say that doctors in any way inevitably misuse this power. Nevertheless there is considerable potential for patients to feel overawed by their own feelings and anxieties, and to leave the surgery completely unheard. We will be returning at a later stage to this theme of power in the therapeutic relationship and its importance in the whole process of getting well.

Drugs and the culture of power

If the issue of power within the medical establishment and between individual doctors and their patients is an important one, there is also a further power issue to be considered within the culture of medicine. Alongside doctors and their patients there is a further player, the pharmaceutical industry. Some would claim that the chief beneficiaries of modern medicine and its enormous costs to governments and tax payers are not the individual patients but the companies who manufacture and distribute drugs. While we should be cautious of such claims, it is clear that both governments and the medical profession experience the power and influence of the industry. The quoted expenditure on the promotion of drugs is said to exceed by three times the amount spent on research. Thus every GP may be 'wooed' to prescribe certain drugs, by offers of free gifts, payment to attend conferences, and other inducements. Although most doctors would not dream of behaving unethically, the pressures are certainly there.[1]

Where power is expressed in so much expenditure it is hard to see that objective clinical judgment will always be preserved. Just as there is an ethical issue to be addressed in the way that power is exercised by the medical profession as a whole and by individual doctors, so there is also an ethical problem about allowing an industry to spend so much on persuading its customers to use its products. The continuing promotion of drugs would not happen unless the companies concerned believed that they were being rewarded for their effort and expense. Clearly if individual doctors had all the evidence that they needed on which to base expert clinical judgment, no one would submit to drug company persuasion and the whole system of promotion would be a waste of time. But the pharmaceutical industry does not believe it to be so.

Conclusion

In this chapter we have looked at the culture of orthodox medical science and the medical profession, and some of their underlying principles. We have seen that in spite of its power and pre-eminence in our Western culture, medicine has a context within the history of philosophy and ideas which, in principle, makes it open to criticism from those who do not share some or all of its presuppositions. The issue of concern that arises from the very success and prestige given to medicine and its practitioners by our society is the issue of power. It was noted that the profession does not only have to address the issue of power in its own territory; it also stands in a relationship with, arguably, a still more powerful partner—the drugs industry. Relationships which involve power always raise ethical issues and it is to these we will find ourselves returning.

CHAPTER 2

Beyond the Medical Model: Mind–Body Healing

In the last chapter we explored some of the conventions of orthodox medical thinking and some of the philosophical ideas that undergird methods of treatment.

We noted how medically trained doctors are more at ease with the diagnosis and treatment of physical symptoms than with looking for environmental or psychological causes of illness. Indeed, according to the strict principles of medical science, the mind is separate from the body. When disorders of the mind occur, as we shall see in the next chapter, they are to be investigated by an entirely separate branch of medicine—psychiatry.

That the human mind might have a role in the origin and healing of a physical illness is a hypothesis which some doctors prefer to leave on one side. From a common-sense point of view mind and body are connected, but bringing them into a close connection makes the understanding and treatment of an illness more complicated. Thus they are kept apart as long as possible.

In this chapter, we are going to look at the findings of some medical researchers who have identified the part played by the mind in both the disease and the healing process. Such research leads us to look for a more conscious harnessing of the mental capabilities of human beings to promote healing of the body— healing which may rest on unexplained facets of the human being, but which has had documented success.

The placebo effect

One of the most striking aspects of the relationship between doctor and patient is that the mere giving of treatment is often sufficient to promote healing, regardless of whether it has any relevance to the condition. In the days before effective drugs were available, a bottle of foul-tasting but chemically inert pink medicine might be dispensed by the doctor, and not infrequently its effects for healing were dramatic. Delivered with all the authority and confidence of the healing professional, this produced an expectation and confidence in the patient that would play a crucial part in the process of getting well.

The fact that harmless substances may sometimes effect healing in patients is something that has to be taken account of in the work of researching and establishing the effectiveness of new drugs. The 'placebo' effect, the possibility that an inert substance may effect healing, has to be carefully addressed in every drug trial by what is known as the double-blind test. Neither doctor nor patient knows whether the substance given is chemically inert or a sample of the drug under test. This is to exclude from the mind of the patient an expectation that the drug will effect healing. The placebo effect can be seen to be of the greatest significance to anyone interested in the mechanisms of the mind in the healing process.

Research undertaken in the 1950s[2] suggests that about a third of patients are helped by the administration of a placebo and the effect is not limited to one group of conditions. There is one particularly striking case[3] of a woman who suffered from severe nausea and vomiting. Nothing given her seemed to work. Then the doctors involved gave her a 'new and extremely powerful wonder-drug' and within twenty minutes the nausea had disappeared. The wonder-drug was, in fact, syrup of ipecac, a drug designed to induce vomiting. Somehow the expectation or 'faith' that the drug would relieve the nausea persuaded her brain to set up a response in the body to regulate the nausea.

The placebo effect is not just operative with the administration of drugs. In the 1950s a fashionable operation on the heart[4] involved tying off an artery in the chest as a way of relieving chest pain. Surgeons became enthusiastic about the operation as patients reported great improvement in their symptoms, and measurements on electrocardiograms seemed to bear out these subjective impressions. Some surgeons, however, doubting the physiological basis of this improvement, set up a test where a placebo operation was offered and compared it with the genuine procedure. When the placebo operation proved to be as effective for the patients as the genuine operation, the whole technique was abandoned after no less than 10,000 operations had been performed.

Another phenomenon long noted by doctors is linked to theplacebo effect. During World War II, American soldiers in the Pacific who were wounded badly enough to need repatriation only needed medication in a minority of cases. The expectation of leaving the front line for home gave meaning to these injuries so that they could even be welcomed. Somehow that sense of relief was more than enough to distract the soldier from his pain. In other words, the perception of pain varied with the state of mind of the person experiencing it. The literature on the placebo effect is full of examples of the way that, when the mind is aroused by faith, expectation or hope, the brain seems to effect healing, or at any rate considerable relief from symptoms, through mechanisms of its own.

It would be wrong, as I hope our examples have made clear, to see the placebo effect as 'merely psychological'. The results can be real and often permanent. Those who have studied the process are not clear about exactly how it works but clearly the brain, when aroused in a particular way, can mobilize very powerful self-healing and pain-relieving mechanisms. These factors are probably at work every time we go to see someone, whether it be a friend, doctor, psychologist or priest, that we believe can help us. Faith in a person, a healing procedure or God can release something in us that is potentially health-giving and physically transforming. Such a well-attested mechanism in the healing process as this should perhaps be affirmed more, and used in conjunction with other therapies. Also welcome would be a greater effort by health professionals to understand the exact mechanisms involved in this process.

Mind and Healing

In the literature on mind–body healing there is one particular story that is much quoted about the power of the mind to help the healing processes of the body. It concerns Norman Cousins, an American journalist who was suddenly taken ill after a particularly difficult trip to Moscow. He was left crippled by an arthritic condition that left him almost totally immobile. His doctors declared his illness to be both progressive and incurable. In the middle of his pain and helplessness he decided that, with the help of his doctor he was going to take charge of his illness and its cure. He had read about the negative effects of stress and the chemical changes such stress has on the body so he decided that he was going to tackle his illness with positive emotions.

Before embarking on his plan he had stopped taking huge doses of aspirin and butazolidine along with other painkillers and sleeping tablets. The part of his self-treatment that is most remembered was his 'laughter cure'. He set up in his hospital room a cine-projector, and with this he would watch old *Candid Camera* films. He found early on that ten minutes of laughter would provide two hours of peaceful sleep. He also found that the blood sedimentation rate, a measure of arthritic activity, dropped significantly after each laughter episode. The other main plank of his self-healing programme was to take large intravenous doses of vitamin C. The healing process continued steadily and he was able once more to take up his job at the *Saturday Review*.

Cousins remained unsure about which part of his treatment, the laughter or the vitamin C therapy, was the most important in his getting well. A significant aspect of the story was that Cousins decided to take responsibility for his own healing. That decision, in turn, aroused in him powerful energies for healing in his mind that neither he nor his doctors had previously known.

Norman Cousins' story has not ended. Thirty years after his illness, several hospitals in Canada and the USA have introduced laughter into their arsenal of weapons against cancer and other illnesses. A story in a Canadian newspaper in 1993 reported that a hospital in Calgary has a 'humour cart', with videos, books, games and toys. The plan is also to have a hospital-wide comedy channel on closed-circuit television. Before his death in 1990, Cousins himself lectured widely on his experiences and was invited to join the medical school at the University College of Los Angeles as a faculty member of the Department of Psychiatry and Behavioural Sciences. Clearly the academic world took Cousins and his reflections on his illness seriously, and as a layman he has been allowed to be part of a movement to understand the interaction between the immune system and the brain.

Today we find an increasing understanding among researchers about the way the brain uses chemicals of all kinds to communicate with the rest of the body. Out of the research which Cousins himself sponsored came some new understanding of the way that laughter can, in fact, increase immune cells while simultaneously decreasing cortisol, a hormone that suppresses the immune response. Other research has been carried out into the pain-suppressing chemicals released by the brain called endorphins. These seem to be activated by the brain through the pituitary gland in situations of stress when the so-called 'fight or flight' response is provoked. There are numerous accounts of individuals injured in sport or battle who have not felt the pain until long afterwards. The brain was apparently blocking awareness of pain until the crisis was over.

A further interaction between mind and body is found in the way that individuals appear to thrive far better in satisfactory social environments. It has long been noticed that bereaved people not infrequently die of a 'broken heart'. People who move away from familiar surroundings, leaving behind friends and family, also suffer from more health problems than those who continue the social networks that they have built up over many years. Again, the mechanism by which individuals in good social circumstances remain healthier than those who are isolated has not been well understood. But in the late 1970s there was some sustained study of the physiological effects of bereavement. In one patient who had suffered bereavement, it was possible to measure lower activity in a particular white blood cell, known as a T-cell, that attacks foreign invaders. This decline in immune function lasted for up to fourteen months, after which time levels had returned to normal.[5]

The stress of a bereavement, by affecting the immune system, can result in a whole variety of different complaints from flu to cancer. It would seem that there are links between the mind and the immune system even though the mechanism has still not yet been completely described. One hundred years ago the famous French sociologist Emile Durkheim, in his study of suicide, noticed that Protestants committed suicide more frequently than Catholics. After excluding many other factors he reasoned that Catholics were less likely to kill themselves because they had greater social networks than Protestants. For the first time social factors were seen to be components of the health of society.

There is a great deal of current research about the effects of diet and heredity on the incidence of heart disease. Some of the research will be looked at in Chapter 4, but one important piece of work was conducted in the 1970s among Japanese people living in America[6]. It had long been known that nationals who live in Japan have rates of heart disease one-fifth of the level of Japanese people living in the United States. It had been thought that when they emigrated to the States and adopted Western lifestyles their rates of heart disease would shoot up to equal American ones. But two epidemiologists, Michael Marmot and Leonard Syme, identified a group of Japanese immigrants in California whose rates of heart disease were similar to that of their own people back in Japan.

In their analysis, Marmot and Syme discovered that the difference between this group of Japanese and other ones in America lay in their social networks. Both groups had equally high levels of cholesterol, through eating Western food, and had similar high blood pressure and smoking habits. But the Japanese who preserved their Japanese way of life, medical practices, cultural events, and political and social gatherings were far less susceptible to heart disease. In short the research indicated that social stability was perhaps the key factor in the maintenance of health, even more important than diet and smoking. The mechanics of how social support affected the functioning of the body through the mind were again not fully understood. But this piece of research, along with religious teaching through the ages, suggests that love, community and unselfish attention to others are good for you.

In our attempt to understand how our minds and relationships affect our health for the better, it is worth reflecting for a moment on the way that the human race developed and flourished because of its ability to co-operate and work together with other members of the same species. Just as the infant needs to stay with its mother or another lactating adult for its biological survival, so social co-operation, especially through the human family and the sexual bonding that takes place within it, is a crucial aspect of healthy human functioning. People need people for the maintenance of their health. A study of the health of individuals after the experience of divorce showed that trauma was a health hazard equivalent to the smoking of twenty cigarettes a day[7].

As another example, the longer life span of women may be partly attributable to the fact that they are better able to make bonds of friendship outside the home than men, bonds which continue to support them during the experience of widowhood. Men certainly appear to suffer more when bereaved.

A Swedish experiment examining the effect on health of social isolation among the elderly compared two groups of older people[8]. One group was given a socially active programme with time spent on botany, art, music and song. This in turn resulted in a threefold increase in social activity between staff, residents and outside people. The other group did not participate. At the end of a six-month period it was found that the group involved in the social enrichment programme had increased in height, perhaps from improved posture or actual changes in bone structure. Levels of anabolic hormones, which protect the body from stress and generally build up health, had also increased. The other group had decreased in height.

There is much more that could be included in this section about the negative effects of stress on bodily functioning, and the way that hard competitive ways of life sometimes result in sudden death. Most people know within their own circle of friends an individual who has destroyed his or her health by living life under enormous levels of tension and stress. But I have chosen to focus here on the ways the mind can affect health positively rather than negatively, though clearly the mind can work in both directions. The title of a book published in the early 1980s, *Mind as Healer, Mind as Slayer*, sums up the double-edged activity of the mind acting through the brain.

There are two words that sum up so far the positive ways that the mind can actively produce health for an individual—faith and love. These two words also carry religious associations, and the health-promoting aspects of both these attitudes are used by many in the religious healing endeavour, Christian and otherwise.

Hypnosis

In planning a presentation of the different cultures and modes of healing, I had wondered in which section hypnosis should come. Should it be regarded as a therapeutic technique, aligned to psychotherapy, and thus concerned with mental healing? Or is it a practice that demonstrates the interaction between mind and body in its entirety?

Although hypnosis was used by Sigmund Freud in his early career for the treatment of mental illness, even he used it only as a method of accessing deeper levels of the mind prior to a return to consciousness. More obvious, even to the non-expert, is the apparent way that hypnosis enables the mind to act on the body in bizarre and totally unexpected ways. Thus hypnotized people in response to suggestion see and hear things that are not there and apparently feel physical sensations which have no basis in reality. The mind is obviously acting in a very powerful way, creating realities of its own. In this we can see connections with what was said earlier about the power of the placebo, the capacity of the mind to be suggestible to the outside influence of a healing personality. Thus a discussion of hypnosis belongs to the present discussion of this chapter—the capacity of the mind to affect the body for good and ill.

To speak of an individual being 'suggestible' at once raises ethical questions about this therapy. The relationship between a patient and therapist using hypnosis, for whatever reason, would appear to be one of considerable closeness and dependency. Commentators have observed that hypnotic techniques are used not only in one-to-one relationships but also when powerful leaders manipulate crowds. Writers in Europe are alert to the part played by crowd hypnosis in the political history of their countries and the techniques practised by such leaders as Hitler and Ceausescu.

When hypnotic methods are used for the purpose of manipulating crowds there is a dangerous and powerful mixture at work. When Christians use this combination of techniques the dangers are not automatically lessened. The potentially unethical use of hypnotic techniques in so-called 'Gospel preaching' is too little examined by Christians themselves. While they are ready to criticize hypnosis as an unchristian activity when practised in an individual context, there is too little readiness to notice that a different form of the same technique is sometimes brought into the church itself without any awareness of its potential dangers.

At this point we need some further working definition or understanding of hypnosis that will enable us to examine further the implications of its use for healing. It is difficult to find any agreed definition in the textbooks. The one we will settle on here may not satisfy experts in the field but it will help us begin to make sense of the technique in the healing process. For us, hypnosis is a state of trance with complete or partial suspension of normal conscious awareness; the mind attains a state of hyper-suggestibility so that the will of another person can easily take over the hypnotized subject. Normally unconscious faculties of the mind are simultaneously released to become active. In its claim to be able to activate mental abilities which can affect physical mechanisms in the body, hypnosis has an effect very much like the placebo considered earlier in this chapter.

It is unclear whether the first reputed practitioner of hypnosis, Franz Anton Mesmer, in the Paris of the 1780s, actually practised what we would call hypnosis at all. Mesmer's techniques were based on his theory that animal magnetism passed from one person to another, much as a magnet exerts a magnetic force. This animal magnetism, understood to be a quasi-electrical life-force, often sent his patients into convulsions rather than the peaceful state of sleep-like trance which we associate with the technique today. Mesmerism was, however, developed by his successors and survived both as a therapy and as a form of entertainment, particularly in the United States.

As we shall see in Chapter 5, mesmerism or magnetic healing fed into the mind techniques of healing developed in nineteenth-century North America. As a therapeutic technique, hypnotherapy was used by Freud before being elaborated into his theory of psychoanalysis. Today it has been rediscovered as a serious therapeutic method, and it continues alongside stage hypnotism which television brings to the living rooms of millions of people. The accomplishments of ordinary people under hypnosis are puzzling, but this writer at any rate has no reason to suppose that either stage hypnosis or hypnotherapy are not genuine phenomena.

We need to say more about the capabilities and achievements of the mind released through hypnosis. The first, most striking facility is the mind's ability to screen out pain so that surgical procedures can be done without anaesthetics. Another, often promoted by stage hypnotists, is to see things that are not really there. The mind can clearly hallucinate in a hypnotic trance. A further capability, which caused some embarrassment to Victorians but is little investigated today, is the ability of the mind under hypnosis to achieve clairvoyant insight. In one investigation in the mid-nineteenth century that would be condemned as unethical today, a schoolteacher, Alfred Wallace, used his pupils as test subjects and, to his surprise, one of them reacted to whatever bodily sensations Wallace felt[9]. Every prick or pinch was felt by the hypnotized boy. It was as though hypnosis uncovered a group consciousness.

I include this anecdote because it may illuminate puzzling phenomena that sometimes occur in Christian healing contexts when charismatic healers appear to be given direct awareness of the complaints of individuals in the congregation. Hypnosis may be able to reveal a mechanism of mind that can link people together, both in their consciousness, and in states of health and ill health. What scientists refer to as 'mass psychogenic illness', a simultaneous outbreak of disease among hundreds of people with no apparent physical identifying cause, may also be an example of this process or mental capacity at work.

There are also some recent clinical studies on the role of hypnosis in activating healing in the body. In one study in the USA in 1959[10], a group of fourteen patients who suffered from warts were hypnotized and told that the warts on one side of the body would disappear. Within a few weeks the warts on the treated side of nine of the patients had significantly regressed but not on the other side (although one patient did achieve the disappearance of the warts from the untreated side six weeks after the first side had improved). Another experiment in Japan studied thirteen high school boys who were known to be highly allergic to a particular plant[11]. Under hypnosis they were touched with a harmless plant but told it was the poisonous plant. All the boys demonstrated some degree of skin disturbance, believing that they were in contact with the poisonous plant. When the poisonous plant was used and they were told that it was in fact harmless, eleven of the thirteen showed no response to the plant.

In spite of these and other findings, hypnosis or hypnotherapy is not normally used to treat physical illness. It is, however, routinely used for individuals with a psychological disturbance of some kind, or who may wish to give up smoking or lose weight. But from what we have seen, its potential may go further in the task of effecting healing.

There are many contexts in which words, suggestions and symbolic gestures have a powerful effect on suggestible minds, both for good and for ill. Hypnotic phenomena are thus not restricted merely to the use of hypnosis by a trained therapist. Some crowd settings as well as certain types of relationships may cause some individuals to be influenced and affected by methods which are hypnotic in their effect. In short, hypnosis offers us a clue for understanding the mechanism by which some individuals achieve remarkable changes in their physical or mental state. I would even suggest that, as a phenomenon, the hypnotic effect may be far commoner in society than many of us realize.

Conclusion

This chapter has concentrated on looking at some scientific studies of the way that the mind interacts with the body to promote genuine healing. The examples given have not come from religious or spiritual contexts. But in our examination of these examples we have been led some way along a path which predisposes us to find similar episodes in more obviously religious settings, that are neither unlikely nor unbelievable. There are clearly many mechanisms of healing at work in a human being. The new research on mind–body medicine opens us up to new possibilities previously thought impossible according to the conventional wisdom of the scientific world-view. Individuals appear to interact with others in a health-giving way; people can be opened up in a crowd setting to what can be a physically transforming energy. These phenomena are difficult to understand and may seem rather dangerous and best ignored. But this work will claim that, far from being new, most of what we have encountered in this chapter is well known to traditions which have pursued healing outside the modern scientific paradigm. To these traditions I will return.

CHAPTER 3

The Healing of Mental Distress and Psychotherapy

In the first chapter we looked at problems of physical illness and methods designed to deal with it. We noted that a conventionally trained medical doctor will learn methods of diagnosis and treatment based on a particular theory of the functioning of the human body, a theory which is linked to the philosophy of dualism between body and mind. In the second chapter we explored some research which qualified these traditional ideas and which stressed the unity between body and mind. We also explored the importance of these findings for the treatment of physical illness. The research findings that were summarized came mostly from work that was conducted according to the disciplines of academic life.

In short, apart from the speculations in the section on hypnosis I tried not to stray too far from the world-view that scientifically trained people would recognize as being part of their culture. All the first four chapters of this book will respect the presuppositions of this scientific culture, with its insistence on the need for properly conducted tests of all hypotheses before they can be accepted.

When we turn to the area of therapy concerned with the healing of mental distress, however, we find that we are forced to go beyond scientific fact and hypothesis into theories which do not have the same strict laws of evidence and proof to support them.

I do not propose to spend any time on the area of mental health treatment which involves drugs or other physical methods. There are several reasons for this. In the first place, the administration of drugs and electro-convulsive treatment (ECT) for mental illness is an area of considerable controversy and it would be hard for an unqualified person to offer an informed view in this difficult area, particularly in a short summary. Secondly, in the overall selection of material for this book there is a general preference for describing healing methods with involve the empowerment of patients; thus I am drawn in my consideration of the treatment of the mentally sick to look at the techniques of psychotherapists.

Psychotherapy, the broad term to cover the work of clinical psychologists, psychoanalysts and psychotherapists, is an exploration of the individual's inner world of feeling and experience. The tools and methods through which this world is explored belong to intuition and sensitivity, areas with which the explicit world of scientific fact is not easily associated. Psychotherapy lays claim to seek genuine healing through co-operation with the mind's own regenerative faculties. It focuses on the inner world of the experience of the client and attempts to free him or her from what may be a crippling failure to function effectively among other people and in particular situations.

While it is forced by its very nature to explore areas of subjectivity and thus be subject to constant revision and change, it is broadly accepted as a valid therapy by the vast majority of people in our culture whether or not they are scientifically trained. Few people, not even patients, are bothered by the wide variety of 'schools' into which the discipline is divided. If a particular therapist is trusted, most people will also accept and trust that therapist's particular training and the insights that flow from it.

A conceptual framework for psychotherapy

Individuals seek help from mental health professionals when they find themselves unable to cope with the stresses of life; for in this failure there is suffering and distress. Such inability may be caused by constitutional factors, or by a brain disorder or defect; or there may be some experience of trauma from the past, like sexual abuse, that make people liable to a sense of defeat and demoralization. When overwhelming distress takes over in their lives, and is perceived to be caused by an internal psychological conflict, individuals often seek out another person to help them. In psychotherapy, an attempt is made to offer clients a new perspective on the events that are proving so hard to cope with, and through it a fresh strength to carry on.

All people have within them a continuing need to make sense of the world, and it is from our past experience of life that we acquire a sense of coherence and stability for the present and the future. When our experience of the world is and has been reasonably stable, we can form wholesome attitudes which are rooted in positive life affirming experiences from the past. For instance, adults who as children enjoyed satisfactory relationships with their parents will have a better chance themselves of seeing their spouses not as parental substitutes but as people in their own right. A mature rather than a dependent marriage relationship will normally have greater stamina in the face of adversity.

However, some attitudes we acquire are based not on positive experiences but on negative and fear-provoking events in the past. Thus our response to stressful situations in the present may sometimes evoke distant but distressing emotions from the past. For example, many of us from time to time have the experience of meeting individuals who remind us of people who used to bully us when we were children. We find ourselves all too easily responding to them with the physical or psychological defensiveness of the original relationship. Such occasional flashbacks to distressing incidents are counterbalanced for most of us by the recall of positive, life-enhancing emotions, also from the past, which continue to nurture us and our appreciation of people in the present. Thus rational attitudes to present events can exist alongside irrational ones.

Unfortunately, irrational ways of responding to life's events are not always recognized by the conscious mind. Past experiences with all their attendant emotional 'baggage' can remain in an individual's psyche to be experienced as an eruptive force in the present, causing disabling inner conflict and distress. It is about such situations that psychotherapists are concerned. Some attitudes may have been formed around negative experiences and a client or patient may consequently react to the world, either occasionally or permanently, with a sense of impotence, bewilderment or despair.

The understanding of some areas of trauma is still relatively new. For example, it is only in the last decade or so that we have begun to understand the fearful havoc wrought on proper adult functioning by sexual abuse in childhood. Such kinds of trauma with their attendant negative emotions can cause an individual to cower in a metaphorical corner, resistant to any movement forward or to the possibility of new experiences in life. Sometimes the symptoms of distress are disguised by an individual who is able to put a good front on problems within. But real suffering lies just below the surface, taking away the joy and spontaneity of life and its richness.

Common features

Among the many schools of psychotherapy certain common features stand out, and we shall dwell on these common features, rather than attempt to offer a preference for one particular approach. The first thing that therapy offers is a personal relationship with a therapist who is prepared to accept the sufferer and show some genuine concern for his or her well-being. The therapist offers the promise of standing by the client however difficult the problem, and however outrageous the past or present behaviour.

Secondly, there is a special place to which the client goes, a place of safety, a setting in which to be true to self without fear.

From a religious perspective, 'pilgrimage' is involved, a moving from the ordinary to the special place of healing and support.

Thirdly, the therapist will seek to provide a rationale or 'myth' which will enable an individual to understand the symptoms and causes of distress. This is what is known as the 'Rumpelstiltskin factor'—the naming of what was formerly hidden and unknown. To describe such a naming as the creation of a 'myth' is a way of saying that the explanations of illness will vary according to the world-view of the therapist. These world-views will depend on the particular culture or philosophy of the therapist and the choices made out of the many 'myths' or conceptual frameworks on offer. We will be looking further at some of these world-views in the next section.

The final feature of psychotherapy is the procedure offered to remove symptoms, whether it be relaxation, hypnosis, emotional flooding or the reliving of emotionally distressing experiences.

In this section, psychotherapy has been seen as a discipline based less on science than on philosophy. Attempts to prove that one procedure is better than another have even failed to prove that the outcomes of individuals in therapy are better with trained therapists than with lay persons. The literature has spawned articles and books which seek to show that the whole enterprise is an enormously expensive industry which serves the burgeoning army of therapists more than the suffering people they seek to serve. The American experience of individuals having therapy because of a failure to find meaning in life suggests that, for some at any rate, psychotherapy is a form of self-indulgence and a way of buying attention and company.

Whether or not people accept criticism of psychotherapy, it is nevertheless true that therapists from Freud onwards have caused a fundamental revolution in the way ordinary people look at relationships in families, among friends and in the work place. For example, the sadistic punishment of children in the name of

Christian discipline that was practised extensively in the last century is almost totally outlawed today. Child abuse is still widespread but at least it is not practised in the name of some godly higher principle. Psychotherapy has also provided an enormous amount of insight to ordinary people who want to bring up their children and manage their marriages with a degree of wisdom and insight. Moreover, in seeking to serve others with problems in a helping, friendly way, a little understanding of the principles of psychotherapy goes a long way in obtaining a detached view of the issues.

This percolation of the culture of therapy into ordinary human situations produces an increased understanding of the dynamics of human relationships, and gives the discipline as a whole as great a triumph as the practitioners themselves. The entire culture of family life in the West, in spite of its many failures, may be far more healthy than that experienced two generations ago. Insight into sexual matters, the possibility of creating discipline without fear and cruelty, and the possibility of men and women being relaxed and physically affectionate towards their children have all made the families of today far more free, by and large, than they were a hundred years ago, for instance. A return to the repression, both sexual and emotional, that obtained in the last century would not be a return to wholeness or health for the majority of our population. Nothing so far contradicts the idea that psychotherapy, both professional and lay, promotes a culture that can be described as healing in the full sense of the word.

Models of the mind

We have already indicated that therapists have recourse to a wide range of therapies, each based on a considerable number of theories about the way the mind operates and finds its full and healthy functioning. Two models in particular have traditionally exercised a great deal of influence in the thinking of all psychotherapists: those of Sigmund Freud and Carl Jung. Their influence is such that few therapists operate without being followers to some extent of the theories of one or other of these great masters. Most psychological models can trace their origins back to one or other of these two pioneering minds, even though their ideas have been considerably altered over time, particularly Freud's.

It would now be useful to spend a little time considering these and other models of the mind, noting that they remain models that lack the precision of scientific experiment. But as models or maps they remain useful as long as the practitioners do not insist, as has often happened, that the human individuals before them have to fit the theoretical strait-jackets of these models. Psychotherapy, as we shall see, can all too easily move from being a compassionate, caring therapy into a form of tyranny by the healer over the sufferer. Making sure that vulnerable people in search of healing fit the theories and models of the healer's reality is a temptation known to healers of every culture.

My criticisms of Freud are therefore criticisms of any individuals who, in the setting of a healing relationship, use power to prove the theories they hold. The reality of the individual before them is always more important than any theory or model, and people who seek healing will always transcend the models of reality into which healers try to place them and their experiences of distress.

Of the two thinkers Freud is probably more important than Jung, even if much of the edifice he constructed has been much criticized and modified today. Freud took up observations from many of his predecessors about the unconscious workings of the human mind and saw the importance of bringing these to the surface and integrating them with the conscious mind. He recognized that there could be states of conflict between the 'ego', the aspect of the personality in touch with the external world, and the instinctive urgings of the 'id'. He is best remembered for his theories about the development of the child and his formulation of the so-called 'Oedipus complex', with its sexual connotations. According to Freud, 'only sexual wishful impulses from infancy are able to furnish the motive force for the formation of psychoneurotic symptoms'.

Freud claimed to discover in the repressed memories of adults a sexual longing in young children for the parent of the opposite sex. In projecting sexuality on to small children Freud seems to have passed by the possibility that children themselves, particularly girls, were the sexual victims of their own parents on some occasions. Some of the most chilling accounts in psychoanalytic literature are the records of Freud using his power as the expert helper to coerce his vulnerable patients into the truth of these 'wishful' theories. The account that Freud himself gave of the treatment of a girl he calls Dora—he insisted on 'interpreting' her descriptions of sexual harassment by a male friend of the family when she was only fourteen—is an account of emotional barbarism. In Freud's interpretation, Dora in some way became the instigator of the assault rather than the victim. Other detailed accounts of work with patients confirms that the detail of some of Freud's theories about the functioning of childhood are based on the flimsiest of evidence.

Of course, theories and speculations about the sexual life of young children are in themselves fairly harmless as long as they remain speculations. But the moment they become part of the professional standing of the theorizer and need to be proved to protect a reputation, they become dangerous and harmful.

Some therapists are seen to exploit the weaknesses and the vulnerability of their patients, but the particular misuse of power that Freud, and no doubt many of his followers, are guilty of is the protection of their maps of reality which, as noted above, is a temptation for healers of every culture.

Indeed, many psychiatrists in the past labelled misfits in society as mad and in need of institutional protection. My old parish in Herefordshire possessed a large Catholic convent for the 'care' of girls who in the years up to the First World War were considered to be in need because they were 'in moral danger or likely to fall into moral danger'. No doubt these girls were the spirited ones in the family who were unruly and risked opposition to convention. Their exasperated parents found some psychiatric doctor who would agree with them, and they were shipped off to Hereford and deprived of personal freedom, never to leave the convent for any purpose for fifty years, and spending all their lives running a laundry.

In the nineteenth century the crass, authoritarian histories of psychiatry were also chilling. We should not therefore be surprised that Freud himself continued the tradition of authority which put theory and dogma above compassion and common sense. But in addition to the issue of the abuse of power, one final point needs to be made. In all his voluminous writings, Freud never developed a satisfactory understanding of 'wholeness' in the functioning of the ordinary human individual. To him, the goal of life appeared to be a discovery of some compromise between the gratification of blind instinctual energy and the need to meet the requirements of society represented by the super-ego. There seemed to be no sense in fulfilling a spiritual vocation or even in finding the meaning of love above and beyond sexuality. Freud's system certainly became a powerful myth or philosophy of the human mind, but its lack of a vision of wholeness now disqualifies it as a satisfactory or complete model of healing for today.

By contrast, the philosophy of Jung does present a vision of the unity of the psyche. Like Freud, Jung saw the human personality as a multi-tiered system, with the conscious ego afloat, as it were, over both the individual and the collective unconscious of the human race. He described how psychic energy from the unconscious welled up into the ego or persona, while some elements of the individual's potentiality were repressed to form a 'shadow'. Because of this repression of opposing or unacknowledged aspects of the psyche, Jung believed that the individual could only be fully realized when the repressed elements were released and integrated with the conscious elements of the mind. The goal, he said, was the achievement of 'individuation'—a balance of energy between the forces within and those without, taking into account the personality type of the individual, whether 'introvert' or 'extrovert'.

Readers of Jung who come from a spiritual tradition will note that he saw within human beings an intrinsic drive towards wholeness which was understood very much in spiritual terms, as a need to reconnect with the Absolute, or God. One could claim that, in so far as individuation and wholeness are the same thing, spirituality, prayer and healing are all connected in Jungian thinking. Certainly, many people from Christian and other spiritual traditions have found Jung a rich source of inspiration and guidance for their practices of healing. The somewhat esoteric insights contained in his massive *Collected Works* will always remain a quarry for those who share Jung's belief that the human mind is a vast reservoir of mystery, creativity and potential.

A third map of the human person which has much that is attractive about it is the humanistic client-centred psychology of Carl Rogers. The picture he offered was of the human personality moving out from its limited or damaged past 'toward constructive fulfilment of its inherent possibilities'. For Rogers, the task of psychotherapy was to set free this potential and for this certain things would be needed: first genuineness and openness in all relationships (including psycho-therapeutic ones); secondly acceptance or 'unconditional regard'; and thirdly, empathetic understanding.

For a long time this non-directive, affirming approach to counselling has had great appeal, and in its warmth has seemed very close to the Christian ideal of love. But in its optimism and apparent unawareness of the issue of evil within individuals, it is perhaps not an approach that can be accepted uncritically. The notion of 'human potential' is one that we shall meet later on in this work but we need to feel a certain caution when the fulfilment of individuals is stressed without any apparent acknowledgment of personal responsibilities to others. Carl Rogers himself would probably not be proud of the way that his ideas have been taken over by a section of what is known as the 'New Age' movement, with its cultivation of experience for its own sake beyond the ties of society and ordinary human responsibilities.

A final model or approach that we need to look at briefly is that of Gestalt. This is a style of counselling first developed by Fritz and Laura Perls in Germany, and later at the Esalen Institute in California. The German word defies an exact English translation but it has the meaning of 'meaningful organized wholeness' which, by implication, many people fail to achieve. In Gestalt therapy, individuals are encouraged to become aware of their immediate feelings and responses, including those contained in their body language. The process, normally conducted within a group, involves 'owning' and 'sounding out' of feelings which would otherwise be lost. As a style of therapy this can be fairly forceful and may be as uncomfortable for some clients as it is liberating for others.

Conclusion

This survey of psychotherapy is inevitably incomplete but it tries to affirm the overall 'healing value' of approaches which offer a human relationship of trust and stability with which to face the reality of mental distress. We have mentioned the part played by the 'myth', the interpretative framework of the therapist, in making sense of the world-view of the patient. But we have noted how such myths or maps can become vehicles of power abuse and oppression when they are so much part of the professional identity of the therapist that they are imposed on clients,like a political or religious ideology which cannot be questioned. Psychotherapy, like any other training or professional system, needs a measure of self-discipline and humility if it is to offer genuine healing in a suffering world.

CHAPTER 4

Food as Poison, Food as Healing

From time to time the health education bodies exhort the public about food: to eat less of certain foods and more of others if we wish to preserve good health.

We are, according to the experts, eating too much animal fat, salt and sugar, and too little fresh fruit and vegetables. For reasons discussed in the first chapter much of this advice is ignored. People take comfort in the apparent disagreement among the experts, not noticing that, were there to be a major revolution in the eating habits of this country, a vast and profitable food industry would have to make an expensive readjustment. So there will always be experts disagreeing with each other, taking advantage of whatever research claims suit their particular corner of the food industry.

It is not my purpose here to take sides on such issues as the respective benefits of butter versus margarine or vegetarianism versus meat eating; rather I wish to look at the broad issue of food as a determinant of health, both negative and positive. In our society the issue of food for health has produced a recognizable sub-culture and for this reason we need to look at it and see it alongside the other healing sub-cultures addressed in the book.

Food intolerance

Individual intolerance and allergies to particular foodstuffs are becoming more widely recognized in our society. Controversy will, however, continue to reign over claims that individuals can obtain a considerable measure of control over their health through the avoidance of certain foods. The problem, in short, is that even if individual sensitivity to a foodstuff is a factor in ill health, it is not something that can be uncovered by a short consultation in a doctor's surgery. It requires a great deal of effort to discover whether intolerance to particular foods is involved in an illness, followed by yet more effort subsequently to avoid those particular foodstuffs. Nevertheless, if certain foods do cause ill health, there are enor-mous implications for the health of many people. It also returns to individuals a measure of controlling their treatment, together with a welcome alternative to drugs and other potentially unpleasant treatments. It is, moreover, significant that food is implicated in many chronic conditions that are not amenable to more than 'management' by conventional treatment.

A few years ago I met up with a friend who had been stricken by ankylosing spondylitis, an arthritic condition of the spine which is extremely painful and disabling. He had followed a diet which excluded red meat, alcohol and dairy products and had received total relief from his symptoms. Every so often he would slip back from the diet and have a glass of red wine. This would cause some of the pain to be felt again. It was as though he had still got the disease but it only manifested itself when particular foodstuffs were present. In the summer of 1990 this same friend rowed with his family down the River Thames to London from my parish of Lechlade.

Also in my present parish are a number of older men who have controlled their symptoms of osteoarthritis through diet alone. Food sheets are exchanged and mutual encouragement is offered. Nothing leads me to suppose that either the illnesses themselves or the relief obtained are anything but genuine. But alongside this group are others I have met for whom the idea of taking some control over their illness by trying a diet is total anathema.

Food avoidance does seem to be a genuine part of healing even if it has not entered the mainstream of medical thinking. Doctors have, however, known for some seventy years about allergic illnesses including eczema, asthma and hay fever. These are often caused by environmental pollutants, such as the house dust mite, animal fur, pollen and certain chemicals. In our house a constant battle is fought against the dust mite and its droppings; otherwise sneezing and even asthmatic wheezing result.

It is when we leave these recognizably allergic illnesses and symptoms that controversy begins. The orthodox medical view is that such illnesses as rheumatoid arthritis and Crohn's disease are unlikely to have their symptoms triggered by particular foods. Additional claims that foods can cause such things as depression, anxiety and even psychosis are not acceptable to mainstream thinking.

Resistance to the possibility that particular foods are able to cause a whole variety of illnesses in susceptible individuals is, in part, caused by the philosophy of medicine that we looked at in the first chapter. The germ theory of disease gave medicine a cause-and-effect model to explain the origin of particular diseases.

By contrast, knowledge about food intolerance is vague, and sensitivities are extremely difficult if not impossible to pin down. Unlike allergy diseases, where specific tests indicate the activity of an allergen, food intolerance operates according to no known mechanism. It cannot be repeated in two different individuals because the intolerances of each person are different. If someone gets better after avoiding eggs or milk products it could be the result of coincidence or the universal catch-all, the placebo effect.

Dr Doris Rapp, a paediatric allergist, resisted the idea that foods could cause hyperactivity in children for fifteen years. Finally she witnessed a dramatic improvement in a five-year-old after putting her on an elimination diet. Three days later the teacher of the child rung up to ask what drug the child was on! But in the profession as a whole, the question of food intolerance remains one of belief or disbelief. Those who believe in it practise it with good results, while those who don't believe continue to find support for their position! Thus for the foreseeable future patients who have complaints for which food intolerance may be a factor may normally have to look outside the medical profession for help and advice.

Although support for the idea of food intolerance is not widespread, some trials have been carried out. One trial at Epsom District Hospital[12] involved fifty-three patients with rheumatoid arthritis. It was conducted with all the safeguards of a controlled trial, with the examining doctors not knowing which patients were on the diet and which were not. The researchers were impressed when three quarters of the diet group, all of whom eventually went on the diet, claimed to feel 'better' or 'much better' than at the outset. Another trial at Northwick Park Hospital in Middlesex had a less successful outcome[13]. Eighteen patients were studied over six months with no statistically significant improvement. However, the test was flawed because wheat, a commonly implicated food in arthritic diets, was not excluded. A further important study of food intolerance in migraine sufferers was carried out at Great Ormond Street Children's Hospital in 1982[14]. Of the eighty-eight children in this double-blind trial, 93 per cent benefited from the diets.

The link between the mind and the eating of particular foodstuffs is the greatest area of controversy. Most of the interest in this field can be traced back to a book published in 1976 by Dr Richard Mackarness, Not All in the Mind. He described the results of dietary change in a patient called Joanna who had suffered from the most horrifying mental symptoms over seven years. After a five-day fast during which she showed 'a very marked improvement in her condition', she was tested with some of the eliminated foods to see her reaction. The symptoms returned with certain of the food stuffs and a particularly virulent reaction was noted with regard to coffee. A psychiatrist expressed surprise at the results but could not fault the way the test had been carried out. Dr Mackarness has since retired and now lives in Australia; one hears less today of the work that he began.

No one has yet mounted large-scale studies of the extent to which food intolerance might be implicated in mental distress such as schizophrenia or depression, but clearly even one successful double-blind trial means that this approach deserves a more thorough examination, even though it goes against cherished ideas of the causes of mental illness. Drug therapy for the majority of mental conditions seldom appears to provide actual healing of the condition. A sustained attempt by the medical profession to research the question of food intolerance in mental conditions would seem a productive avenue of research, even if it were to lead to relief for only a minority of patients. The avoidance of certain foods as a treatment would have much to commend it; certainly it would avoid the problem of side-effects, a problem which seems to plague the use of drugs in cases of mental illness.

The hypothesis that food intolerance may cause various chronic illnesses is one whose day has not yet arrived. But I believe that it is only a matter of time before those who follow this particular approach are heard. A more sympathetic audience will then be gained among the public and the medical profession at large. Quite apart from the correctness or incorrectness of this approach for individual patients, the avoidance of certain foods demands a co-operation from the patient which gives back to him some control or power over his condition. The patient can decide to do something which may help the illness and thus raise morale. Even if hopes are dashed later, can we really say that such participation in the treatment of disease is misguided?

Hope for the eventual healing of an illness is something that should not be taken away from a patient lightly. Hope which is given by actions that individuals can take themselves is a particularly important kind of hope, a hope based on personal power and responsibility. Such hope is a kind of faith; and faith, as we saw in Chapter 2, is an important prerequisite of healing.

Food as medicine

It was Hippocrates who said over 2,000 years ago, 'Let food be your medicine'. There is today no shortage of literature and research to suggest that certain foods do have important preventive qualities and in some cases curative effects.

One area of contemporary discussion centres on the effects of certain kinds of fat contained in our food which affect the functioning of cells within the body. Many bodily processes such as blood clotting and inflammation are controlled by hormone-like substances collectively known as eicosanoids. Two particular kinds of fat make these eicosanoids. They are known as the omega-3 fatty acids, largely obtained from marine sources, and the omega-6 fatty acids which are derived from vegetable oils and animal fats. It seems that the wrong proportion of omega-6 to omega-3 fatty acids can cause havoc in the body, leading to heart disease and cancer. Likewise a concerted attempt to correct this imbalance between the two fatty acids can lead to relief in various degenerative conditions such as ulcerative colitis and high blood pressure.

A Danish study in 1988 suggested that more schizophrenics get better in countries where there are high levels of the important fatty acids in the diet[15]. More recently, *The Times*, reporting on a conference in Florence in June 1994, described the work of Dr David Horrobin and his research on essential fatty acids[16]. The drug company of which Dr Horrobin is chief executive, Scotia Pharmaceuticals, is researching a manufactured compound containing two fatty acids which have been shown to benefit patients who have had operations for heart disease. A compound called EF13 is to go on trial on the basis that it will show impressive results against certain forms of cancer, as well as cells infected with HIV. Drugs based on compounds contained in our food can and do make a major contribution to the fight against disease.

Garlic is another important food believed to have almost miraculous qualities, both in preventing illness and in treating long-term disease. It seems that garlic may help clear blocked arteries and prevent further damage. One particular trial that tested garlic on patients with cardiovascular disease was conducted in India[17]. A cohort of 432 patients suffering from heart disease was divided into two groups. One group was given garlic daily as a morning tonic and the other was not. After one year there was no difference in the death rate between the two groups, but after two years the death rate among the garlic eaters was 50 percent lower than that of the non-garlic group and after three years it was 66 percent lower! Garlic apparently contains at least fifteen antioxidants that may neutralize artery-destroying agents.

The fatty acids in sea fish and garlic have been shown to have a positive effect on health. Other research exists to indicate the benefits of walnuts, fresh vegetables and other foodstuffs. These are just some areas where medical research appears to confirm the health-giving properties of particular foods. As a whole, diet-based therapy either as food avoidance or as food supplementation may provide a unique and special place in the search for health.

Vitamins and minerals

Research in the early part of this century into certain illnesses such as beriberi and rickets resulted in the discovery of the substances we call vitamins that occur naturally in food. Since those early days, recommended daily allowances (RDAs) of these vitamins have been established for people to take through their diet. These RDAs are based on the quantities needed to avoid deficiency diseases.

The new thinking is that greatly increased quantities of some vitamins may be helpful and even necessary to prevent and sometimes treat certain illnesses. In Chapter 2 we saw how Norman Cousins chose to consume large doses of vitamin C to fight his arthritic complaint. Such use of vitamins is not infrequent in the treatment of diseases of various kinds. Research continues, particularly in the United States, into the disease-preventing and healing properties of all the vitamins and minerals that have been shown to be active in the human body. The pattern of this research seems to be that hypotheses about vitamin and mineral efficacy are often first aired in 'alternative' or fringe literature, and then adopted by a body of orthodox medical opinion. From there, results of trials and consequent evidence about the use of vitamin supplements tends to be mediated to the public by the press.

It is interesting that while many adults in Western countries are taking vitamin C supplements, deficiencies continue to occur among certain sub-sections of the population — especially the institutionalized elderly, one group for whom extra medical attention might be expected. There are many claims for vitamin C—the prevention of cancer, cholesterol-lowering properties and the speeding up of wound healing. If even a tenth of the claims for it were true (and all have been the subject of clinical trials), one would expect to see supplemental doses given widely, particularly for those in institutional environments where the style of cooking so easily destroys this vitamin in the food.

However, vitamin and mineral supplementation, despite all the claims made for it, is unlikely to make a great deal of progress in our society for the foreseeable future. Most conventionally trained practitioners still cling on to the original research which established the recommended daily allowance of each vitamin and mineral needed to prevent actual deficiency. For this they claim that a well-balanced diet is sufficient to provide all our needs. Therapeutic doses of vitamins and minerals make little sense in a medical culture geared to the treatment of disease through drugs and surgery; it should also be pointed out that some vitamins can be toxic in high doses. Nevertheless, a fair proportion of the general public, by their use of supplements, have rejected what they think is out-of-date information.

In the end, the question about whether supplements and therapeutic doses of vitamins work is not the only issue. The real issue is that there seems to be a clash of interests between a powerful drugs industry which makes profits from treating illness and an alternative one supplying supplements to an increasing number of people. The reason for taking these supplements is the laudable attempt (whether misguided or not) to take some responsibility for keeping healthy and certainly the research to support people in this desire is impressive. An acceptance of responsibility for one's health through vitamin supplementation may act for some as a placebo. Either way, health is maintained and governments should be grateful for attitudes that make good health a reality for many people; the health of even a small group of people is a valuable asset for any country, however it is achieved.

Conclusion

The subject of mineral and vitamin supplementation completes this rapid survey of the way in which food and the avoidance of it may play an important part in the promotion of health. The research undertaken in the last ten or twenty years is extensive, but it requires a particular kind of motivation to search out the information and act on it. Too many of us are reliant on those health professionals who are oriented towards the treatment of disease rather than the exploration of methods to prevent it. An interest in the topics outlined in this chapter takes one into a different health culture—the culture of self-empowerment rather than the culture of passivity combined with deference to experts when things go wrong.

Health and healing are once more seen to a considerable extent to depend on the individual's readiness to take responsibility for his or her own health, to make informed and intelligent decisions about what is right. We need that fundamental shift in attitude that

moves us from being 'patients' on a doctor's list—expecting at some
point to be ill—to becoming partners with all health professionals
who are concerned to teach us about our bodies, minds and spirits.
It is such knowledge, combined with a motivation to act on it, that
will do much to move our health service from being disease-centred
to becoming health-centred.

CHAPTER 5

The Background to Alternative Methods of Healing

The first four chapters of this book have explored the notion of healing from the broad perspective of mainstream culture. Some of the healing methods so far described are controversial, but those who have researched them would maintain that they fully accord with the conventions of academic life.

This next section of the book concentrates on what might be summarized as systems of healing based on alternative cultures. Those who hold to these systems are aware that such healing is not part of mainstream medicine, or at any rate that it has roots some way from the historical traditions of Western thought.

In view of the rapid advance of conventional medical science over the past fifty years, the rise of alternative healing systems in Britain and North America has taken many people by surprise. Inasmuch as such systems are considered at all, they are perceived as a cultural reaction to the traditional medical practices of the West which are perceived to lack 'soul', and which rely heavily on technology and other impersonal methods.

'Alternative medicine' is one strand of these new healing systems,and it has been welcomed by at least one group within the medical profession. There is, however, a dislike of the description 'alternative', as some of the techniques are regarded as 'complementary' to the practice of conventional medicine. Those medical practitioners who welcome some of the methods of alternative medicine would therefore prefer the title 'complementary medicine' to describe the particular techniques that meet with their approval. But it may be appropriate to hold on to the title 'alternative' for all the systems of healing, medical and otherwise, that are described in this chapter. The reason for this is that each of them emerges out of systems of thought which are alternative to orthodox Western culture. It is these background systems of thought to which we now turn.

The religious and metaphysical background in the USA

In the early nineteenth century, the United States of America was a young, confident country, and the energy with which it created new institutions was seen in the wide range of religious, political and social movements founded in the first century after Independence. The 1830s were a particular period of energy for new ideas and institutions. In the religious sphere emerged the Mormon Church, the Shaker movement, and the Revivalist movements of the so-called Second Great Awakening under Charles Grandison Finney. At the same time, systems of healing such as homeopathy and mesmerism were also making their appearance in defiance of the medical *status quo*.

Homeopathy originated in Germany, but it acquired a wide following among the urban upper classes in the United States, in conscious opposition to the crude medical practices of the day which, as we have seen, focused on assaulting the body with crude and largely unproved treatments rather than working with its innate powers of recuperation. Homeopathy followed the principle that 'like cures like'. A much diluted dose of a substance that produced symptoms similar to those suffered was given to the affected patient. To quote the founder of homeopathy, Samuel Hahnemann: 'The healing power of medicines depends on the resemblance of their symptoms to the symptoms of disease.' It was not long, however, before the procedure became aligned with the currents of metaphysical or religious thought that were widely current in the 1840s. Hans Gram, the pioneer of homeopathy in America, was reported to have 'led the way to a wider and deeper knowledge of the relations between body and soul, the human and the divine, the transitory and the permanent, than can be entertained by purely materialistic researches'.

Mesmerism, which we have already encountered in Chapter 2, was brought to North America in 1836 by Charles Poyen, who described himself as a Professor of Animal Magnetism. In his lecture demonstrations, he was accompanied by an assistant who was particularly adept at entering the trance state. He also enlisted members of the audience to whom he explained that he was going to heighten their body's supply of animal magnetism so that they would not be responsive to their surroundings. The sense of theatre in these performances estranged Poyen from the medical and scientific communities, but many flocked to his performances in the hope of a cure from physical ailments. Healings indeed took place, according to contemporary newspaper accounts—healings from such afflictions as rheumatism, back disorders and liver complaints. Also reported were various clairvoyant feats, including inexplicable communications between the operator and those who had been mesmerized about unspoken thoughts.

Poyen returned to France in 1839, but by 1843 there were two hundred 'magnetic healers' in the city of Boston alone. The mesmeric state seemed to point to a 'sense in man which perceives the presences and qualities of things without the use of... the external organs of sense'. When patients were in touch with what a British mesmerist, Chauncy Townsend, called 'the inner source of feeling', healings could occur spontaneously. Such levels of consciousness had much in common with religious mystical states and it is not surprising that an understanding of healing which stressed a spiritual or metaphysical cause came to be widespread in American thinking of the period. This was in contrast with the conventional medical insistence on physiological or psychological agents for disease.

A further element which fed indirectly into American alternative healing systems was the speculation of Emanuel Swedenborg, who lived in the eighteenth century in Sweden. An eminent scientist of his time, he also wrote extensively on the theme of the spiritual essence beneath the literal meaning of Christian doctrine. Swedenborg appealed to those who wished their Christianity to possess a spirituality which went beyond its church manifestations.

Swedenborg's beliefs can be summarized as a system of thought that popularized the idea of correspondence or harmony between physical and spiritual realities. His God was a reality to which people could be attuned, an indwelling cosmic force. Swedenborg explained the universe in the manner of ancient Greek religion, with different dimensions interpenetrating one another. The object of each dimension was to establish contact and harmony with that above. Thus the physical body, he believed, could achieve inner harmony by being attuned with the mind, the mind with the soul and the soul with the order of angelic beings. Such harmony between the different dimensions created the possibility of healing both emotional and physical disorders. Swedenborg's ideas came to North America at around the same time as mesmerism, and to- gether these theories helped to give unorthodox medical thinking there its particular characteristics.

This background of American thought, particularly from the 1830s and 1840s, will provide a means of understanding two important religious systems of healing which we shall be examining in Chapter 7, Christian Science and Spiritualism. This same background has also percolated through to influence what can broadly be described as 'New Age' healing, discussed in Chapter 8. But here the concern is to see how these ideas illuminate the original background of two of the most popular alternative healing systems of the nineteenth century, chiropractic and osteopathy.

From metaphysics to physical healing—chiropractic and osteopathy

Daniel David Palmer, the founder of chiropractic, was born in 1845 and began his professional life as a practitioner of magnetic healing, an intuitive method of healing by touch. In this he would be close to many practitioners of today, often described as 'healers', who treat through a combination of psychic abilities and the capacity to create a close rapport with their patients. Palmer himself reported taking on the pain and symptoms of some of his patients. But, true to his culture, he held with other 'magnetic healers' that the principle involved in this therapy was the manipulation and enhancement of 'animal magnetism' in the patient, which would affect the course of the illness.

One idea that Palmer pondered was that the flow of magnetism might be blocked by obstructions along the spine. He discovered his particular technique when treating a deaf neighbour, Harvey Lillard. Lillard had, according to his own account, become deaf after exerting himself in a stooped-over position. Palmer then felt along his back and found an unusual lump in the vertebra. He applied pressure, the bone slipped back into place, and Lillard could immediately hear again. Palmer then developed his new philosophy of healing, which held that vital energy flowing via the back to all the organs of the body sometimes became blocked and needed clearing by manual pressure on any misplaced vertebra.

Palmer developed his ideas in conformity with his spiritualist and mesmerist background, describing the human organism as the vehicle of a spiritual principle or energy he called 'Innate' and which in turn was 'part of the Universal Intelligence, individualized and personified'. Palmer's son continued this metaphysical emphasis within the teaching of chiropractic until his death in 1961. Such a principle had the advantage of giving the theory of chiropractic a simple understanding about the human organism both in health and in disease. The extent to which the contemporary chiropractor has retained this theory will be seen in the next chapter.

The other main healing system of the nineteenth century was that of osteopathy, invented by Andrew Taylor Still. Like Palmer, Still was brought up in a world in which healing was closely associated with religious and metaphysical ideas. He set himself up as a magnetic healer in 1874, having turned his back on a rudimentary medical training with its dependence on the harsh treatments of the day.

In his practice of drugless medicine, Still drew on a further tradition of nineteenth century therapy, that of the bonesetter. Again, like Palmer, he found an intuitive way through manipulation to heal conditions that the medicine of the time was unable to help. By 1892 he succeeded in founding the American School of Osteopathy. In this school, Still's principles were taught alongside more conventional medical techniques ,although Still resisted this at first. Like Palmer, he had dwelt on the metaphysical aspects of his discoveries and was anxious to see osteopathy as a discipline alongside theology. He saw his healing technique as releasing the divine intelligence that is manifest within the physical order.

In its metaphysical and religious traditions, America has been a potent source of inspiration for many alternative ideas of healing. Our understanding of the contemporary culture of alternative medicine would be incomplete without an awareness of the enormous religious energy of this particular period of history. The next chapters will look at how many of these themes have penetrated various strands of thinking that are popular today.

Beyond the materialistic model of the human body—the contemporary background

We have looked at the USA in the nineteenth century and seen how, just below the surface, much of the official, orthodox view of both scientific and religious reality was under challenge. The same underground challenge to the dominant world-view is also a feature of our present century. In the first place, this counter-culture has found inspiration in the findings of higher physics; in the second place, it looks to the cultures of the traditional societies of the East, both Chinese and Indian. The combination of these ideas forms another stream of inspiration for those who wish to see the issues of health and healing in a completely new way.

Conventional thinking about the universe and its system of working is based on the discoveries of Isaac Newton in the late seventeenth century. He taught people to see the universe as consisting of solid objects which interacted with one another in a mechanical way. Human beings were no exception to this overall pattern. But this Newtonian method of thinking had to be qualified, first of all by the discovery and investigation of electromagnetic phenomena. Michael Faraday and his colleagues described a 'field' which created forces when another object was present. In the early twentieth century, Albert Einstein undermined the Newtonian model even more fundamen-tally with his insights about the inextricable connection between space and time. More importantly for a new paradigm of the human person, Einstein indicated the interchangeability of matter and energy.

In the 1920s, research in physics began to unravel still more extraordinary features of the universe when examined at subatomic levels. New insights were gained about the way that matter cannot be regarded as 'solid'. Matter did not consist of solid blocks as common sense and observation suggested. Rather, phenomena at their most elemental level were better explained in terms of their relationships and their interconnectedness. One writer, Henry Stepp, summed it up by saying: 'An elemental particle is not an independently existing unanalysable entity. It is in essence a set of relationships that reach outward to other things.' This pattern of interconnectedness pointed to a new way of seeing both the universe and the individuals that live within it.

Teachers of a healing paradigm that involves the use of energy fields or auras will claim that their insights fit well both with the wisdom of traditional religious teaching and with the insights of modern physics. The latter enable them to claim that there is nothing inherently improbable about the human body possessing subtle energy fields. Moreover, they claim that these auric energy fields may interact negatively and positively with those of others.

This kind of language fits in with ancient Hindu tradition and its reference to a universal energy called *prana*. This energy is held to be the breath of life, and it is the manipulation of this energy that is the aim of yogic practices. Chinese traditional thought also spoke about the life force or Qi, which contains two opposite forces, the yin and the yang. Health depends on the balance of these two forces.

The concept of auric energy, in terms of a quasi-physical radiance around an individual, is not unknown to the Christian tradition. In Eastern Orthodox spirituality, one goal of the mystical quest is the vision of the 'uncreated light' that was seen around Christ on the Mountain of the Transfiguration. The idea that spiritual illumination can be experienced as a quasi-physical radiance around an individual has long been part of Orthodox thinking. In particular it is expressed in iconic art, with its representation of radiance around the pictures of the saints.

Many alternative healing systems, both medical and non-medical, use the concept of energy flow as an important part of their rationale. It is important to note that research into these energies and their power for healing has been reported in the pages of parapsychological journals for some time, although little attention has been drawn to the fact until quite recently.

One particular research partnership was set up in the 1960s between Dr Bernard Grad, a researcher at McGill University in the United States, and a healer named Oscar Estebany. The experiments set out to show whether Estebany could heal mice with surgically created wounds. Those mice who were 'treated' did, in fact, heal at twice the speed of the others—the treatment, administered by Estebany, was to hold their cages for fifteen minutes twice daily for fourteen days. Other experiments showed that healing could inhibit the growth of goitre in mice that had been given a drug affecting the activity of the thyroid gland. These experiments, however bizarre, clearly indicated that some energy transfer was taking place which had nothing to do with 'suggestion'.

There are many therapists who would say that such experiments fitted into the world-view required by their particular techniques. Energy manipulation or energy transfer underlie the theories of numerous alternative therapies, some of which we will be encountering in later chapters. Those who use this kind of language would claim that it is the only coherent form of language which expresses the phenomena that they are dealing with. The new paradigms of modern physics and the experiments of Bernard Grad and others may be indicating that a scientific world-view is at last catching up with phenomena that have been known about in many parts of the world for thousands of years.

Holism and healing

Earlier in this chapter, I said that at least one section of the medical community is taking seriously the paradigms that underlie alternative healing systems. This group of doctors have created a style of medicine which they call 'holistic medicine'.

Holism as an idea goes back to the book *Holism and Evolution*, by Jan Christian Smuts. In this important study on the philosophy of science Smuts pointed out the inappropriateness of using the language of traditional physics in respect of living systems. His argument can be summarized as stating that the whole is greater than the sum of its parts., and to talk meaningfully about living organisms is to refer to them as wholes rather than collections of parts. Thus holistic medicine looks at the whole human organism, including its physical and emotional environment, when treating disease.

Practitioners of holistic medicine are fully conscious of the findings of modern physics, particularly the stress on the interconnectedness of matter revealed at a subatomic level. They also take seriously the metaphysical insights of Eastern thought and are not afraid to talk about healing energies at work in the processes of disease and healing. In short, many of those practising holistic medicine are prepared to enter imaginatively into the paradigms of other healing cultures in an attempt to bring health to patients.

The work of promoting holistic medicine requires skill not only in scientific areas but also in philosophy, history and culture. Of all the healing cultures looked at in this present work it is the only one that has, I believe, successfully crossed the barriers between traditional and unconventional modes of thought. For that bold imaginative achievement, holistic medicine deserves a very high regard even if not all people, at the end of the day, share its enthusiasm for the strange and the exotic.

Conclusion

Many alternative healing systems feed off the broad pattern of ideas that have been outlined above. When we come to them for the first time, some of them seem strange and esoteric and have little in common with a common-sense world of reality. But we live in a world where the old models of reality do not, in fact, always seem adequate to account for the immense complexity of human experience. There is a value in having our attention drawn to phenomena which are normally simply ignored by the models of explanation allowed by our culture.

As a Christian, I feel it is only when the widest range of ideas are explored that I can begin to understand where I really belong and what I stand for. It is only when we have travelled widely among contrasting worlds and systems of ideas that we can recognize and value afresh the place we want to call home. But whatever we do call home, we need not reject other differing philosophies outright. It may be possible to grow and find our convictions deepened in a continuous interchange with ideas that come to us from outside.

Later in this book we will be examining the distinctively Christian culture of healing. That culture, although possessing a coherence and completeness of its own, does not exist in isolation. It has always existed alongside the very distinct and even contradictory culture of medicine in healing matters. Perhaps Christian healers also need to discover a new way of relating to the cultures, ideas and patterns of thought which emerge from different roots and philosophies. What we have today is a world of many cultures, all clamouring for attention in the world of healing as in many other areas. Perhaps the approach of this book can encourage a generous response to these cultures even where they emerge from sources quite separate and distinct from those we understand and with which we are comfortable.

CHAPTER 6

Alternative Medicine

In the previous chapter we looked at a number of religious and metaphysical ideas which lie behind many of the varieties of alternative healing which are around today. Many of these alternative healing systems have emerged from unorthodox world-views, and thus their treatments should in a real sense be described as 'alternative' to medical science and its methods.

This chapter will look at some of the healing therapies which are normally referred to as 'alternative medicine'. Those examined involve treatment of the body with physical or quasi-physical techniques. A further chapter will look at alternative methods of healing which involve the mind and spirit, and the power of attitudes and mental techniques to affect the course of illness.

In looking at the range of physical therapies which can be loosely described as 'alternative medicine', it soon proves impossible to do anything like adequate justice to the subject in a short chapter. One reference book I have consulted lists seventy therapies which are practised by alternative practitioners. What can be given is a flavour of some of these techniques—homeopathy, chiropractic, aromatherapy, acupuncture, Bach flower remedies, herbalism and reflexology—and how they relate to the background of unorthodox ideas looked at in the previous chapter.

In discussing this selected group of therapies, no recommendations are made about their effectiveness. The important task is to see them within the cultural and philosophical setting to which each belongs. They all appear to be coherent and plausible once people enter imaginatively into the respective world-views of each system of healing, leaving to one side any prejudices and beliefs about what makes human beings either healthy or diseased.

Chiropractic

We have already looked at the historical origins of chiropractic and its founding by David Daniel Palmer. Most modern chiropractors distance themselves from the metaphysical ideas of their founder; rather they involve themselves in the treatment of 'subluxations' or slight displacements of the spinal vertebrae. As long as they treat back pain, they are not considered to be a threat to orthodox medical thinking, particularly as back problems are notoriously difficult to treat by conventional means.

But although chiropractors focus on the gentle manipulation of the back, they do not see their therapy as relevant only to back problems. Their philosophy, as we saw in the last chapter, is to regard much illness as being caused by trapped nerves in the back. Thus chiropractic manipulation is offered as a potential source of healing for a whole variety of complaints, including such afflictions as migraine and joint malfunction.

It is here that I can offer a personal anecdote that may illustrate part of their work. About ten years ago, I visited a chiropractor–herbalist to seek help for my chronic catarrh. I was expecting to be given some herbal remedy, but the therapist said that as I was there he would like to look at my back. I duly obliged and he then asked if I suffered from nausea. I answered that whenever I was under stress, nausea was the first symptom I experienced. I had, in fact, once gone to a GP for some tablets for this some eight years before.

The chiropractor told me that the vertebra leading to the vagal nerve connected with my stomach was slightly out of place and that he would like to put it back. There was a slight click, and I was to realize very soon that my occasional nausea had completely disappeared. It was an unusual experience for me to be healed of something that I had not even told the therapist about!

Looking once more at the question of whether chiropractic is scientific, it has to be said that the therapy has a plausible structure of its own which is quite different from its origins in 'magnetic healing'. Whether that structure of thinking is actually 'scientific' is not easy to say. But I conclude this section with an observation of my own which is based on hunch rather than real evidence. Palmer's success cannot really be accounted for unless he was in some way 'gifted' with his hands. Just as some doctors are drawn to the profession because they are healers in terms of their personalities and presence as well as their academic acumen, so I believe that many chiropractors may possess 'gifts' of touch which their training has enhanced rather than created. Further reflection on 'touch' as a dimension of healing will be found in later chapters. Perhaps chiropractic may 'work' because it involves a combination of gifts—the scientific, the intuitive and the human sharing of love and compassion expressed in touch.

Homeopathy

In the short discussion of the discovery of homeopathy and its development in the nineteenth-century USA, we noted the fundamental principle held by homeopaths that 'like cures like'; this principle is alluded to in the name 'homeopathy', which means 'like disease'. Samuel Hahnemann, the first practitioner of the therapy, had noticed that extracts of the bark of the quinine tree, which relieved malaria, actually caused the symptoms of the disease when he took it. He spent fourteen years researching the principle that a medicine which causes the symptoms of a disease also cures it.

By testing or 'proving' a large number of substances that were able to produce symptoms similar to genuine illness, Hahnemann and his successors built up a *materia medica* that was in radical contrast to conventional treatment. The controversial, and to medical science, inexplicable aspect of the treatment was the fact that the remedy given was so dilute as to be almost non-existent. How could an active substance have any effect when it was diluted to one part in one hundred million?

Until recently, little attention was given to this question and many people were interested only in whether the remedies actually worked. More recently, however, a mechanism identified in quantum physics has been suggested as the one by which homeopathy does indeed 'work': namely, that the substance has left in the dilution an 'energy field' which is sufficient to act on the organism.

Within homeopathy, there is a strong sense of the 'intelligence' of the human body and its efforts to find its way back to harmonious balance or homeostasis. Symptoms are not regarded as enemies to be suppressed or liquidated; instead they are to be worked with as a way of dissipating the energy of the illness. A homeopath will always have a strong sense of the whole functioning of the individual, and for some practitioners this will include a religious dimension. To quote George Vithoulkas, a practising homeopath: 'Health on the mental plane is freedom from selfishness, having as a state complete unification of the person with the divine, or with truth, and whose actions are dedi-cated to creative service.' It is hard to take issue with the sentiments of this statement.

Bach flower remedies

The remedies of Dr Edward Bach are an example of the principle that healing is sometimes a matter of human intuition rather than the application of cold reason. Bach originally trained as a pathologist and bacteriologist just before the First World War. In his dissatisfaction with orthodox medicine, he switched to homeopathy. He became increasingly interested in a patient's emotional state and the importance of treating that area of individual need.

The flower remedies to which Bach's name is linked are the result of an extraordinary process whereby flowers were handled and their properties for healing were discerned by a process of intuition. The particular flower chosen for its healing properties would then be placed 'on the surface of water, in a plain glass bowl in full sunlight for three hours' before the liquid was bottled. Dr Bach left behind him after his death in 1936 a metaphysical basis for explaining the healing properties of his remedies. His explanation was that the flower waters produced had the 'power to elevate our vibrations, and thus draw down spiritual power, which cleanses mind and body and heals'.

We have seen that a climate for this kind of reasoning exists among those who believe that harmony between the body and higher spiritual realms is a prerequisite for health in its fullest sense. But this religious, metaphysical reasoning makes little sense unless one has already become predisposed to it. In fact, the flower remedies and the metaphysics behind them might have been quietly ignored by this book, but for the fact that they have appeared to help people known to me who would otherwise not regard themselves as outside the common-sense view of the world.

One is left puzzled by this particular therapy, but just because proper understanding is difficult or impossible it does not follow that the therapy must be discarded. Of all the alternative therapies it seems to be the furthest away from our ability to understand, yet it may achieve for many people its offer of healing for mental disharmony.

Aromatherapy

Aromatic plants of all kinds have been used both in religious worship and in healing rituals for thousands of years. Frankincense resin, used in Catholic and Orthodox worship as well in some Anglican churches, has been shown to have a psychoactive chemical in its vapour which can stimulate the subconscious. In addition to religious rituals, aromatic oils were also used by the ancient Egyptians for massage, cosmetics and embalming, and it has long been noted that when certain plants or plant resins are burned, different moods can be induced, either of drowsiness or of euphoria. It is not surprising, therefore, to find that the art of healing using the sense of smell should be practised today.

It was in 1937 that a French cosmetic scientist, René-Maurice Gattefossé, coined the term 'aromatherapy' in a book on the subject. Gattefossé had first concentrated on the cosmetic uses of essential oils, but he discovered the therapeutic qualities of lavender oil when he used it to treat himself for burns after a laboratory explosion. The wound healed so completely that not even a scar was left. The practice of giving oils was found to have relevance not only to skin disorders, but also to the strengthening of the immune system and even to the healing of mental conditions as well.

Another Frenchman, Jean Valnet, experimented with aromatic oils in treating wounded soldiers in the Second World War. He, too, saw great improvement in psychiatric patients, particularly in the process of weaning them off the drugs used to treat their disease. His book, *The Practice of Aromatherapy*, is the classic textbook for practitioners.

Two further pioneers should be mentioned: Marguerite Maury, an Austrian, who died in 1967, who pioneered the use of oils in massage; and Robert Tisserand, who is the leading British aromatherapist today and who has done much to give the therapy credibility as far as this country is concerned.

As a twentieth-century therapy, aromatherapy has not acquired the metaphysical theories encountered in other systems. Rather, it has focused mainly on the physiological aspect of smell and its effects on the physical and mental systems of the body. The therapy is 'holistic' in that, apart from its use as an antiseptic, it is generally aimed at toning up the whole central nervous system through massage or by reaching the functioning of the brain through the act of smelling the oils.

The area of the brain associated with smell, the olfactory centre, merges with the limbic system which is concerned with hunger, thirst, sexual desire and also with the subtler responses of memory, creativity and intuition. The sense of smell is also connected with the hypothalmus, the part of the brain that influences the pituitary gland which in turn is in control of the hormonal system. Scents and smells can also affect an individual quite profoundly at an emotional level if they evoke particular memories or associations, either good or bad. Scents do not have to be powerful or even accessible to the conscious mind to affect us. Some tests at Warwick University, Britain[18] have shown that odours so dilute as to be imperceptible to consciousness can cause both emotional and physical responses in the body.

Personal preferences for smell will vary from person to person. An odour that we like will help us more, particularly in relieving stress. These preferences will vary according to age, state of health and natural body scents—pheromones, as they are called. To some extent, then, we need to follow our instinctive preference to select a scent or oil that can help us. In this area the individuality of the patient is affirmed within the treatment.

Where massage accompanies aromatherapy, there is also the important aspect of touch. Although the massaging of oils into the body is thought to boost the central nervous system, any therapy involving touch is likely to involve aspects of healing that are more than purely physical. In massage, touch involves an interaction between two people which can be described as 'intimate' though not sexual. Where intimacy is involved, individuals exchange a human communication that can be described as a loving one. Love in this context may be reaching parts of the personality that purely physical methods may not reach at all. The close attention of the psychotherapist, the touch of the massager, and the love of a healing prayer group may all be reaching levels of personality that need to be reached if healing is to occur. It is not surprising that of the therapies we have looked at so far, aromatherapy has reached a certain acceptability among wide sectors of the caring professions.

Acupuncture

In contrast with aromatherapy, acupuncture can trace its origins back to the dawn of history—even to the Stone Age. Textbooks dealing with acupuncture in China date back to the sixth century BC. Although widely used in China, however, interest in the therapy did not surface into public consciousness in the UK until the late 1950s.

This interest began after a women's magazine ran articles on the use of acupuncture for rheumatism and other chronic disorders, and demand for the addresses of practitioners flooded in. Other therapists hastily took courses, sometimes from books, to meet this new demand. The treatment was, however, still regarded as a form of lunacy by conventionally trained doctors, since the practice of sticking needles into one part of the body to affect a quite separate part of the body made no sense at all in the medical model. It was not until the 1970s that Western observers saw it used for the first time in its Chinese homeland. At that time it was studied for its use in administering pain relief. It was this aspect of the therapy that the Western observers chose to focus on, although acupuncture is used in many other contexts.

The conceptual framework through which acupuncture treatment operates is totally alien to Western ideas. The so-called meridians along which the life force, or Qi, runs are not detectable by any Western instruments. Acupuncture seeks to balance through the use of needles the 'yin' and 'yang', the complementary energy systems of the body. There is a close attention to pulse taking of each of the twelve meridians, six monitored on each wrist. This is a brief process but through it the therapist is able to assess the balance in the body between the energies that flow through the different meridians. Needles are used because they are believed to be able to stimulate the flow of energy in any meridians perceived to be blocked or sluggish. The exact positioning of the needles is a crucial part of the treatment, as they will not affect the energy flow if inserted in the wrong place. Sometimes the process is aided by a technique known as moxibustion, the burning of a cone of moxa (common mugwort) on the needle over the desired acupuncture point.

It has long been known to conventional medicine that the human body has 'trigger points' which respond to pressure or stimulation in relieving pain elsewhere in the body. The mechanics of it have not been understood, and so no use has been made of it in conventional medicine. Some research in the 1970s showed a high degree of correspondence between these points and the traditional acupuncture ones[19].

One variant of acupuncture is the treatment called auriculotherapy, the insertion of needles at certain specified points in the ear to treat complaints in different parts of the body. The ear is believed to possess a kind of map of the body with different points corresponding and relating to all the different organs.

Other conventional research[20] into the effectiveness of acupuncture has shown that it can help relieve not only pain but also inflammation and fever. Those who have tried to fit the existence of meridians into conventional physiological knowledge have been forced to conclude that the body uses 'non-physical properties and energies still largely unknown and uncharted by science[21]'. The fact that this is true should not be a surprise to us. Once we look beyond the mechanical descriptions and understandings of the body known to Western science, we will be forced to take serious account of energy systems that find their meaning only in alternative philosophies and cultures.

Reflexology

A further therapy which is linked to, but distinct from, acupuncture is reflexology. In the same way that auriculotherapy in acupuncture concentrates on specific points in the ear, reflexology concentrates on the way the body's state of health may be reflected in the feet. The basis of reflexology treatment is the stimulation of the feet by massage at particular 'zones' which correspond to diseased or malfunctioning organs.

Reflexology has a history which goes back to the time of ancient Egypt, although it finds its plausibility most naturally in Chinese models of human functioning. This framework of ideas connected with energy flow and meridians does not fit easily into the medical mechanical model, but this therapy should not be disqualified from consideration because of that.

Herbal medicine

Of all the alternative systems of healing that we have looked at so far, herbal medicine is the one that might command the most respect from Jewish and Christian believers. When it says in the Apocrypha of the Bible, 'The Lord hath created medicines out of the earth' (Ecclesiasticus 38:4), the reference is to herbal medicines and not to modern chemical compounds. Indeed, herbal medicines were the only possible medicines available until the advent of synthetic drugs.

Throughout its history, the practice of herbal medicine has been based on a system of trial and error. Particular remedies came to be used for certain complaints because over a period of time they were found to work effectively. The practice, however, came into some disrepute in Britain at the time of Nicholas Culpeper at the end of the seventeenth century, when it became linked to astrology.

The modern science of pharmacology finally overtook herbalism in the last century. It took some of the traditional wisdom of herbalism and used its discoveries to create new products. But, in a very different spirit to that of herbalism, it sought to isolate and finally synthesize the active components of the herbal remedies rather than use the complete plant. The final victory for pharmacology came with the invention of pill-making machines, which meant that the administration of compounds could be a simple, straightforward matter. The use of herbal remedies, by contrast, went into a fast decline as people found them inconvenient to make and saw them as unfashionable.

At one level the modern rediscovery of herbalism is a recovery of instinctive and intuitive elements in the healing process. Sick animals, even domestic ones, will gravitate to plants that can help them recover. When they are ill, chimpanzees in the wild will walk twenty minutes or more to eat the leaves of a particular plant called Aspilia. This contains a microscopic amount of a potent antibiotic which will help them.

Human beings today seem to have lost this kind of sensitivity but it may still be seen in the activities of shamans or healers in more primitive societies. Part of their traditional role is to 'sense' the appropriate herbal remedies for the individuals who come to them for help. It may not be wrong, then, to see herbalism first of all arising out of a sense of oneness with the world.

Although appropriate herbs for healing may first of all have been sought out through a process of intuition, other more pragmatic methods for their choice did emerge later. But in contrast with modern drug methods, the taking of herbs has always been seen as 'holistic', rebalancing the whole body rather than attacking a set of symptoms in the body. Many modern herbalists, while not committed to any particular theory of human functioning, would naturally gravitate to a system which stresses ideas of harmony and the re-establishment of the flow of life energy through the human body. Western herbalists will normally be familiar with the theories of Ayurvedic (Indian), Tibetan and Chinese herbalism, with their distinctive ways of talking about balance and harmony.

Herbalists of today, of course, will have at their disposal not only the experience of hundreds of years of using herbs to treat illness, but also a knowledge of chemistry. Thus they will know, along with pharmacologists, what the active ingredients are in the plants at their disposal. But herbalists will be less enthusiastic than pharmacologists about the way that so many drugs are isolated from the whole plant.

For instance, Rauwolfia, a plant known to Ayurvedic medicine, was used for hundreds of years as a remedy to calm patients down. In 1952, an extract from this plant, reserpine, was promoted as a treatment for high blood pressure. Quite soon, there were alarming reports of the effect of the drug in throwing mentally stable patients into acute manic-depressive states. Other herbal remedies with active chemical constituents also behave differently when they are broken down and used in drug treatments.

Herbalism in many ways links back to the observations made earlier about the healing effects of certain foods. By looking at the patient in his or her entirety, the therapist will seek to find the right herb to stimulate and encourage the natural healing powers of the body, thus defeating the illness. Combining age-old wisdom with the safeguards of modern chemical and pharmacological knowledge, this therapy represents a humane and wholesome extension to the work of medical science and in many areas may provide a safer alternative to some drugs which, by the standards of herbal remedies, are new and untried.

Conclusion

The use of alternative medicines—physical remedies which have roots in systems of thought outside our conventional Western models—has produced great interest in our society. Those who practise alternative medicine claim to respect the wisdom of the human body as it struggles to recover from disease. They value such things as intuition, sensitivity, and the respect for what is 'natural'.

The treatments themselves have been the subject of only a few trials which would satisfy the criteria of modern medicine, but people continue to flock to the therapists who use them. The reason for this may simply be that clients receive from practitioners the time and quality of personal care that is lacking in our technology-driven medical system. Much alternative medicine may indeed be mechanically ineffective, but meanwhile its continuing popularity speaks of a longing by thousands of individuals to return to an older wisdom that has somehow evaporated from our society.

CHAPTER 7

Alternative Religious Healing Systems

In this chapter we move from the physical healing methods of alternative medicine back to a consideration of systems of religious thought, also outside the mainstream, that to a large degree concentrate on healing.

We need to return first to the world of nineteenth-century America. It was there that two of the systems to be examined, Spiritualism and Christian Science, emerged. The ideas and experience that had given rise to the practice of 'magnetic healing' had not only flowed into the physical healing techniques of chiropractic and osteopathy, but had also fed into more explicitly religious organizations devoted to healing.

Christian Science and its historical context

It was in 1838 that Charles Poyen, the mesmerist, visited Belfast, Maine. Among his audience at his lecture-demonstration was Phineas Quimby, a clock maker who was to become the most famous 'mental healer' of the century. Quimby went on to found his own healing practice. His method was to put his associate, Lucius Burkmar, into a mesmeric trance and direct him through clairvoyant means to diagnose the illness of his client.

As time went on Quimby discovered that the clairvoyant process was, in fact, more about tuning into the beliefs, thoughts and feelings of the patients, especially with regard to their illnesses.

This reading of the patient's thoughts and beliefs evoked astonishment and thus tremendous confidence in the therapist. The prescribing of herbs or magnetic passes—the use of gestures to rebalance the 'magnetic fluid'—was coincidental to the subsequent improvements.

Quimby recognized with many other mesmerists that beliefs or 'faith' alone could cure illness, but he went further than this. He claimed that illnesses were themselves caused by ideas and faulty beliefs in the first place. In his words, 'All sickness is in the mind or belief... to cure the disease is to correct the error; destroy the cause, and the effect will cease.'

Quimby shared with other magnetic healers the belief that the source of health was the magnetic fluid or vital force flowing into the body. But Quimby believed that this force, before it reached the body, passed through the mind which in turn acted as a kind of filter. If the beliefs or attitudes of the mind were wrong, he claimed, disease might result. 'Disease is the effect of a wrong direction given to the mind.' Or again, 'Disease is something made by belief or forced upon us by our parents or public opinion.' Thus disease could be tackled by banishing self-defeating attitudes. The individual needed to rise 'to a higher state of wisdom, not of this world, but of the World of Science... the Wisdom of Science is Life eternal'.

These ideas and teachings were taken up by one of Quimby's patients, Mary Baker Eddy. In 1862, she had arrived at Quimby's doorstep a physical and mental wreck. Once healed by him, she dedicated the rest of her life to propagating her own understanding of the cure. Eddy believed it was due to her special reading and interpretation of Christ's healing of the man sick of the palsy (Matthew 9:2–8), claiming that in this passage Christ treated forgiveness of sin and curing of sickness as the same thing. In her frequently revised text, *Science and Health with Key to the Scriptures*, she attempted to bring the ideas of mental healing into a Christian orbit.

It is worth mentioning that the mainstream Protestant and Catholic churches made no moves at all to consider the implications of 'magnetic healing' for their own beliefs and practices, even though such ideas had been deeply influential in American society for some time. In fact, Christian Scientists have never received recognition by mainstream Christians, despite the fact that by Eddy's death in 1910 there were no fewer than 668 separate Christian Science congregations in America alone. But it is not to be wondered that Eddy failed to produce something acceptable to orthodox beliefs when she was attempting something so thoroughly novel without much help. The main divergence with orthodoxy occurred because Eddy insisted that evil, sickness and pain have no ontological reality. Such things, she believed, were the delusions of an erring mind. Everything God created was good.

The task of the healing ministry of Christian Science practitioners was to help individuals to keep their thoughts and minds rooted in the higher laws of God's presence. Christian Science, though much maligned by orthodox Christian thinking because of its unfamiliar and strange metaphysical ideas, has for over a century born witness to a fundamental truth familiar to many Christians. This truth states that prayer and an opening up of the mind and heart to God can affect the course of both physical and mental illness. Had the movement been less tied into and defined by Eddy's text, *Science and Health*, it might well have been adapted and developed into a denomination well respected by other Christian bodies for its pioneering healing work. But in reality it has become a curiosity in Christian circles, locked into a nineteenth-century time-warp of ideas and metaphysics. Few from outside its circle are prepared to make the imaginative journey necessary to translate its considerable, even valuable insights and experiences into a format that has popular appeal in Christian or other healing circles.

Spiritualism

It is no coincidence that Spiritualism as a religious and healing system finds its origins in the nineteenth-century USA. Although the haunting of the Fox family in Hydesville, New York, in 1848 is frequently given as the beginning of this movement, another event in 1843 was perhaps more important. It was in this year that Andrew Davis, who was to become a leader of the movement, was mesmerized by a travelling practitioner, J. Stanley Grimes. Davis proved to be an able trance subject, accomplishing such clairvoyant feats as reading books while blindfolded. Within months he reported that he was in touch with 'mighty and sacred truths' which were being communicated by 'departed' spirits—that is, of dead people.

In his book *The Harmonial Philosophy*, Davis recorded the metaphysical lessons given him by his spirit guides, including Swedenborg. The book explained how, in Davis' view, human consciousness ranged from simple sensory awareness to a higher spiritual state where the mind was in touch with a 'high reality' leading to an 'expansion of the mind's energies'. Healing for Davis, as for mediumistic healers even today, was a matter of attuning oneself to these higher levels of reality and mediating that free flow of energy to one's patients. The actual techniques employed possessed much in common with those of the mesmerist healers of the previous generation.

There is much in both the teachings and techniques of these nineteenth-century pioneers that has come down to the New Age ideas of our own time. Meanwhile the distinctive ideas of the Spiritualists degenerated somewhat from the speculative thoughts of Davis to a somewhat crude concern for contacting the spirits of the dead, often in a show-business type of setting. Table-turning, ouija boards and a large number of parapsychological phenomena were all the rage in Victorian London, and the investigation of these events exercised some of the best minds of the era. While this period of spiritualist activity is not without interest, it remains outside the scope of this study. What is more important is to look briefly at the contemporary practice of Spiritualist healing and note its distinctive place among the cultures of healing today.

For many people today there is confusion in their minds over the words 'spiritual' and 'spiritualist'. The body known as the National Federation of Spiritual Healers (NFSH) is an organization that brings together individuals who would describe themselves as 'healers'. Many of these healers, though by no means all, would claim spiritualistic beliefs, especially in the sense that they believe that they have a 'spirit guide' to help them in their healing work. Harry Edwards, who founded the NFSH, referred to the spirit entities in another dimension who assist the work of healing as 'healing ministers'. Some of these are the discarnate spirits of doctors or surgeons while others come with the names of Native Americans.

The problem for Christian commentators has always been an awareness of the potential dangers of the world beyond with which Spiritualist healers claim to be in touch. Just as we can become infected and oppressed by personalities in this life who can dominate and even enslave us, so there are hazards in opening ourselves up to discarnate personalities from another dimension. To be fair, a study of Spiritualist literature does indicate that the spirits who are claimed to guide the best known Spiritualist healers have all been motivated by what seems to be loving and altruistic behaviour.

Nevertheless, considerable difficulties remain. Communication between the traditional churches and the Spiritualists might have increased understanding of these phenomena, but it has not been good over the past fifty or sixty years and the fault for this should by no means be laid at the door of Spiritualists themselves. A gut reaction on the part of many Christians is that an alleged communication with another dimension (which may, of course, be a delusion) must inevitably be evil. This is not a response that contributes to understanding.

Christians need to be humble about things they do not know, and certainly there is still much that remains to be understood by Christians and others about the claims of Spiritualist healing. Whatever else might account for the life and work of Harry Edwards, who died in 1976 after a lifetime of Spiritualist healing work, there is no indication that he was in any way motivated by a desire for power, wealth and influence.

However, the scandals that have surrounded some Christian healers in the United States show that healing in the name of Christ does not necessarily protect Christian ministry from evil. While this book may take a line of cautious agnosticism on the question of discarnate spirits involved in the practices of many healing personalities, a rather different issue arises for Christians and others who have looked at other less savoury aspects of spiritualist practice. We touched earlier on the Victorian craze for table-moving and ouija boards and it is clear that such practices continue today. If spirits *are* involved in these practices, then such beings would appear to belong to the less salubrious areas of the realm beyond, though some commentators regard the phenomena aroused by occult experimentation as being externalized but fragmentary aspects of the unconscious of the participants, rather than any objective spiritual entities.

But whatever the causes of occult phenomena, certain principles remain true both from Christian and from common-sense points of view. The usual motivation for engaging in occult practice is to gain power, or knowledge, or both. Such chasing after power over other people or seeking selfish advantage through peering at the future is likely to point individuals in a totally opposite direction to that indicated by the Christian faith. For this reason, Spiritualism could be said to involve actual spiritual harm. In short, we need perhaps to make a firm distinction between those who seek spiritualist experience for selfish motives of their own and those who find themselves the recipients of spiritualist communications which they have not sought. At the very least, these latter deserve some understanding and gentleness rather than heavy-handed offers of exorcism from well-meaning but unhelpful bystanders.

In the last resort, talk of spirits, whether by teenagers playing with an ouija board or by a well-known mediumistic healer such as Harry Edwards, may just be a way of describing a set of phenomena that Western culture cannot yet grapple with. The language of Spiritualism may be a kind of mythology to describe the unknowable and indescribable, and our evaluation of it simply as observers will be from its fruit rather than from its theory.

Faith healing

'Faith healing' is a common expression used by many people in society to describe individuals who have a gift of healing touch. The person in the street will use the term indiscriminately to describe people of any culture or belief who use the laying on of hands for healing. Few people actually involved in healing activities, however, will own the expression. Many religious people will certainly distance themselves from the term on the grounds that it appears to reflect a faith in the psychic abilities of another human being. The faith that mainstream religion seeks to promote is a faith or openness towards God, and such faith is not thought to be part of a healing event except in a religious setting.

The word 'faith' in the term 'faith healing' also seems to mean 'imprecise' or 'unpredictable', to contrast it with the conventional treatments of medically trained doctors. In other words, if you seek healing through the psychic or spiritual gifts of a healer, you are choosing an unproven technique rather than the mechanical or proven methods of the doctor. Even many of those outside mainstream religion who practise healing reject the term because of its unhelpful associations with superstition, on the one hand, and its implication that the patient may be dependent on and passive towards the healer, on the other. Each healer within the broad area covered by the term will have a preferred expression, the most popular being that of 'healer' with no other definition.

A 'healer', seen from a Christian perspective, is an individual who operates from the level of a natural, personal, psychic ability in the work of relieving pain and suffering and promoting healing. Some will work from quite sophisticated metaphysical backgrounds, including that of Spiritualism, while others will operate without any theory at all about what they are doing. They only know through pragmatic experience that they have a gift to remove pain and promote healing through touch.

As an example of this latter group, a woman recently arrived at my door who had been to a demonstration of 'healing' at a local centre. The demonstrator had shown the participants how to focus their mental energies through their hands and she directed the group to practise on each other. My visitor found that even after this first demonstration, she was able to cause sensations of heat through laying her hands on her family members (though not her husband) and help them when they had aches and pains. Although not especially excited, she was puzzled about the phenomenon; her visit was as much to satisfy my curiosity as hers.

I felt I was witnessing healing at its most basic level, where the main problem is that we do not have in Western culture a coherent body of language to describe the interchange of energy that is apparently being encountered. As a phenomenon, it probably belongs to the same range of human experiences as that of sensing atmospheres in places and around people without any verbal or visual clues being received. Anyone who has ever experienced anything for which conventional descriptions or explanations have no application will realize that we live in a world where there is a great deal, both within and outside the so-called 'religious' realm, that falls beyond what can be explained. Healing at this basic level begins with something as simple as a mother kissing a child better and extends out to a set of profound but incomprehensible experiences of human communication which lead to healing.

People who practise healing from within the Christian framework of belief and understanding may speak disparagingly of so-called 'faith healers.' Because no one can deny that individuals with a healing gift, at whatever level of sophistication and skill, do sometimes accomplish effective changes in the health of another person, some Christians will feel moved to ascribe the power at work to a malevolent entity, such as Satan. You will often hear faith healers being considered as 'dangerous' or 'demonic' because they are using power without any acknowledgment of its source. The reasoning goes that if it is divine power then the person using it would acknowledge it because such power is unmistakable. But if it is not thus recognized, then it must come from the only other source of spiritual power—the devil, the 'father of lies'. Such reasoning is, I believe, fallacious and unworthy of Christian thinking, however widespread it may be.

A more wholesome approach to this problem is to consider that the phenomenon of healing is part of the natural order of creation, capable of being both good or bad. Like anything else in creation, a failure to acknowledge its true source in God does not make it bad but simply less complete. A gift received in thankfulness is a fuller gift than an unacknowledged gift, but the latter does not become evil because no thanks have been offered. Creation in all its aspects remains good until it becomes the means of deliberate perversion or distortion for some evil end.

There is little evidence to suggest that the vast bulk of 'faith healers' have evil intentions and are thus perverting the goodness of natural creation. If it could be shown that 'healing' is involved in a mother's caressing her hurt child, would this become demonic because it is outside an overtly Christian context? Much work remains to be done in the study of 'faith healing' and indeed Spiritualist healing, both from scientific and Christian points of view. Meanwhile little purpose is served by prejudging the morality of this range of activities which are clustered around the activity we call 'healing'.

A further point needs to be noted about the relationship of the church and 'faith healers'. Historically, the church has looked with extreme suspicion at anyone who has claimed a healing gift. Until very recently only a few forceful personalities such as Dorothy Kerrin and James Hickson have succeeded in obtaining the church's blessing for the use of a natural gift of healing. Most unordained people would have found it wellnigh impossible to practise their gift within the orbit of church life.

The consequence has been that other organizations have arisen who have understood this gift; and naturally gifted people have gravitated towards them and learnt their particular belief systems. No one can really be blamed for unorthodox beliefs when most branches of the church have failed to offer them hospitality or any kind of encouragement or help to understand their gift. The problem continues and many naturally gifted people find their way not into church membership but into branches of alternative medicine, such as massage, where touch is important. Few Christian leaders see this as an issue but one day it will have to be addressed if the Church really wishes to be seen as a healing body where the gifts of all its members are understood and fully used.

Before we leave this topic of healing, we should perhaps consider in what circumstances the activity could become evil. The answer has already been touched on earlier in the book. The morality involved in healing will always centre on the way that we use power. Any ability to affect another person, whether through drugs, meditation or prayer, will involve the use of power: spiritual, psychological or personal. A potential for misusing this power in a way that should be described as immoral is always present. Such immoral abuse of power will be found as much among 'faith healers' as among any other healers, including Christian healers. No one is protected from this evil merely because he or she is using orthodox or theologically respectable methods. Once again, healing is evidently an activity that lays itself open to the misuse of power, the temptation to exploit and the use of another for personal gratification; and in this Christians are not exempt.

Distortions within Christian healing

A fair proportion of Christians who practise healing claim that sickness is commonly caused by demonic or evil forces. Such beliefs create problems for many people, and it is hard to know how far we should take the terminology literally and how far we should see it as a form of symbolic language. The culture of Jesus' time knew the belief in evil spirits and the battle against sickness was sometimes, though not inevitably, seen as a battle against these forces.

For some Christians today these particular beliefs of Jesus and his disciples are taken literally by those involved in healing prayer; thus the majority of healings will involve a combative form of prayer called exorcism. This method of healing, which involves constant battling against demons and evil presences within individuals, raises deep ethical and practical as well as theological problems.

The ethical issues come back to the question of power and the way that it is open to abuse within this type of culture. In any encounter between a healer and a patient where demonic causes of illness are identified, there is an assumption not only that the sick person is powerless before a demon or evil spirit of some kind, but also that the person who names or identifies the spirit has the power and authority to drive it out. Authority over evil spirits is a high power to claim, and the effect of this kind of power may be to create a fearful dependency in the person so diagnosed. The culture where spirits and demons are constantly named is one which is open to fear and exploitation. Such an atmosphere has links with tribal religions where hexing and cursing (in its true sense) are part of daily life.

These comments do not in any way deny that there may be occasions on which it is right for Christians to identify and grapple with the realm of evil. The language and techniques of exorcism and prayer against evil forces are appropriate in a situation where malignant evil is identified. This will occur particularly in the case of an individual who has deliberately sought to be aligned with power from an occult source, whether through satanist ritual or use of an ouija board, though this is unlikely to be an everyday occurrence.

The motive for such activities seems to be the wish to manipulate the world according to the individual's will, through the use of psychic or occult powers. Recent studies on satanist rituals also suggest that participants use them as a way of casting off all ethical constraints, thus sanctioning the abuse and destruction of the innocent and powerless, especially children and women. Whatever happens in such rituals, and here we enter an area difficult to define, the results can be immensely harmful, both psychologically and spiritually. I personally believe that the evil that can erupt out of satanist activities is no less appalling than that seen in wartime when rape, murder and pillage are somehow considered to be acceptable by large numbers of soldiers.

An enormous capacity for evil is latent in many if not most individuals. (I write this when we are remembering the fiftieth anniversary of the liberation of Auschwitz.) As Jesus said, 'it is not what is outside a man that corrupts him but what comes from inside.' Nevertheless, it is appropriate that when the culture of occult evil and satanist belief has created a situation of distress, with possible symptoms of possession, this may be countered by exorcism. What is objectionable is when exorcism is the *only* 'healing' offered to each and every individual for every complaint.

Another serious error in need of continuous refutation and resistance is, I believe, the claim that evil entities worthy of exorcism can enter into a person without their knowledge. Just as conversion to Christ and what is good comes after a conscious choice, so conversion to the way of evil and possession also follows an equivalent decision— a decision, in this case, to seek power and domination over others and the moulding of the world according to the individual's will.

The question remains: where do these ideas of over-emphasis on exorcism and the tendency to ascribe all illness to the activity of demonic beings come from? One theory suggests that the 'house church' movement, a loose alliance of independent/charismatic churches, has influenced Christian thinking with its distinctive ideas of the cosmic conflict between good and evil, rooted in interpretation of the biblical book of Revelation and speculation on the exact timing of the second coming of Christ. According to this teaching, which is now less fashionable but is still known in charismatic circles, Christ is to return to a church which is pure, composed of individuals who are 'demon-free'. As the Pentecostal movement which lies behind the charismatic revival in the United States began with Black leadership, it may have taken into its ethos certain cultural elements from this constituency, particularly the strong awareness of spiritual forces in traditional African cultures which are preoccupied with spirits, good and bad.

These distortions have been included in a section on 'alternative religious forms of healing' rather than in a chapter on Christian healing, because I remain unconvinced that the current interest in demonic causation of illness is a rediscovery of New Testament ideas. Jesus did not interpret every illness as having a demonic cause, and neither should we come to this interpretation until every other possibility has been investigated and eliminated. While any student of Christian healing must take seriously the New Testament insights into the activity of spirits in illness, there is evidence that some Christian groups use this whole way of thinking about illness and healing in a way that demoralizes the sick and manipulates the weak.

If we do choose to say that evil entities cause illness, we need to do so with great care and discernment. Again we come back to the issue of power. Just as the psychotherapist is able to beat down an awkward client by accusing them of 'being in denial', so Christian ministers can, when their teaching is challenged or healing is hard to find, turn on clients and tell them that they are oppressed by demons invited in by some forgotten occult involvement.

The culture of the Jewish world in which Jesus lived was one where evil was identified in terms of personal demons and spiritual entities. Jesus used such language when he spoke of his great struggle with temptation, evil and the powers of darkness. But a twentieth-century emphasis on demonic power to control and dominate humankind and cause mental and physical sickness is a distortion of the New Testament experience and the awareness of Christians through the centuries. This in its extreme form remains a corruption of the Christian faith, and thus has to be placed alongside the other alternative religious cultures of our day.

Conclusion

The phenomenon of alternative religious healing systems in society is, in part, the result of the historic religious traditions in society failing to understand or take healing seriously. The healing practices of 'magnetic healers' in the United States attracted little interest within the church and so movements such as that of the Christian Scientists appeared almost by default. Spiritualism and faith healing filled the gap left by the churches who were unwilling to accept and understand gifted individuals.

Looked at from the point of view of religious orthodoxy, all such alternative healing organizations are found wanting; but our reaction to them should be tempered by a certain humility and a realization that they perhaps would never have needed to come into existence in the first place if the churches had been doing their work of healing. In this chapter the one method of healing that has come under severe criticism is one practised within the church itself. What has been attacked is not exorcism *per se* but the belief that every sickness can be caused by demonic infestation. Such a belief can and does lead to the kind of power abuse possible in all the healing systems described in this book.

CHAPTER 8

Healing and the Spirituality of the New Age

I had planned, in this book, to summarize in a single chapter the beliefs and practices of those involved with the so-called 'New Age'.

However, I soon realized that any attempt to represent the vast range of beliefs called New Age and their relevance to healing would take up a large volume and still leave a lot unsaid. I therefore decided to abandon any attempt at completeness and to focus instead on two approaches to healing to represent New Age practice and its spiritual origins and ideas.

The New Age does appear to have made the concept of 'the spiritual' fashionable to large numbers of people who have not been touched by the traditional churches. This new spirituality remains, as we shall see, sometimes rather shapeless and without personal discipline, but it has entered into the ordinary thought patterns of many people and may appeal to their concepts of healing.

Bernie Siegel and his 'exceptional cancer patients'

The book by Norman Cousins, *Anatomy of an Illness*, which was summarized in Chapter 2, has inspired a large number of doctors to investigate mental attitudes to disease. The main message of that book was that patients themselves can do something to promote healing. They do not have to lie passively waiting to die or to recover.

More recent writings by those who have sought to extend Cousins' ideas have concentrated on the particular challenge of cancer. Here, as Bernie Siegel, a cancer specialist, records in his book, *Love, Medicine and Miracles*, the New Age in cancer treatment dates back only to the mid-1970s.

It was in 1978 that Siegel met the Simontons, a husband-and-wife partnership of cancer specialist and psychologist. The Simontons were leading a workshop on using 'imaging techniques' against cancer. In one meditation, Siegel met George, a 'meditatively released insight from his unconscious', who taught him that he should study the reasons why some patients recover from cancer against all the odds.

Siegel then began his own therapy group. It consisted of patients suffering from cancer; he encouraged them to use all their inner resources to fight their illness, aided by some of the techniques developed by the Simontons. Siegel discovered that up to a fifth of his patients were caught up in a subconscious death-wish; they somehow 'needed' the illness to resolve psychological problems. Another fifth, the ones that Siegel describes as exceptional, refused to play the victim role. Sometimes they appeared to be the awkward patients, refusing to accept passively every test or treatment without having it explained to them; at other times, they demanded to have power and control over their own illness returned to them.

Siegel also learned to question the negative connotations of 'false hope'—he could see that denying hope altogether was not somehow 'better' for patients. On the contrary, he saw that the giving of hope to a patient was an empowerment with definite physical consequences, while denial of any hope contributed to a more rapid decline. Hope also enabled patients to achieve far more with the time left to them than if they meekly submitted to a diagnosis of terminal illness.

A further feature of the group work with cancer patients was the sharing of patients' inner lives. This level of sharing profoundly affected both doctor and patient, making them both partners in the healing process. Too often, Siegel notes, doctors close themselves off from the pain of their patients and this affects their ability to relate to their patients in a healing way. Sharing and caring are a key part of what the doctor has to offer to his patients.

Siegel goes into a lot of detail about the attitudes required and the techniques employed to fight cancer. Patients are taught to meditate, visualize and generally work out new priorities for their lives. One particular message which comes through all his writing is the importance of unconditional love. It describes a way of loving that seeks nothing in return. Many people, in fact, have to learn to love again: they have closed in on themselves because of past disappointment, the need to avoid pain and experiences of betrayal. But in many of Siegel's cases, the advent of cancer is experienced as a catalyst for new life because in the face of the diagnosis everything trivial about life is burned away and there is a new power for making the best of life, which is now perceived as a precious gift.

In my previous book[22], I recalled some words of Lawrence LeShan who ran a workshop on cancer in the summer of 1983 in London. He told his audience that there were three reasons why people wanted to recover from cancer. The first was because they disliked the experience of being ill. The second was because another person in the family needed them, to get through college or to be nursed through an illness. The third reason was because the individual had discovered his or her music for life; they had been brought into touch with their true source of creativity. LeShan stated that the body would not mobilize its powers of healing for the first situation. For the second it would activate them only until the crisis was past. But for the third, the full inner potential for self-healing would be activated. The same creativity is to be found in the discovery of the 'unconditional love', which is an outpouring and sharing of a level of personality which may not have been experienced before the illness.

Bernie Siegel would no doubt be the first to admit that not all his patients survive their cancer. But his books ring with a kind of confidence and strength which resonates well with the mood of self-empowerment that exists in the United States and to some extent in this country. To dismiss them as New Age because they are linked to human potential and self-improvement techniques known in other contexts would be to ignore an important revolution in medical healing. If this were followed through, it could enhance health in the fullest sense of both doctors and patients everywhere.

Dolores Krieger and 'therapeutic touch'

Therapeutic touch is another area of healing with a New Age flavour that has begun to enter mainstream medicine in the United States. Dolores Krieger, a professor of nursing in New York, believed that 'healing' was an ability which could be taught to anyone willing to learn. With the help of Dora Kunz, a professional healer and psychic, her teaching has been shared with tens of thousands of nurses all over the United States. It is never offered as a form of healing independent of medical treatment but as an adjunct to the normal work of hospital care.

The training begins with the premise that anyone can be taught to use this form of healing. Its theoretical basis involves an understanding of energy fields in and around each individual, as we met in the last chapter. Healing comes from the redirection of these energy fields, which have become imbalanced through illness. Because Krieger's work has been conducted in hospitals[23], its value has been measured and thus affirmed in a professional setting. She is, in short, a pioneer, taking something out of the esoteric and exotic realms of psychic healing and bringing it into the mainstream of normal training and hospital practice.

The apparent success of Krieger and Siegel in helping to shift the mood of technological medicine in the United States and to a lesser extent in the UK can be regarded in one of two ways. Some, no doubt, will see their methods as the invidious infiltration of New Age ideas into medical practice, while others will rejoice at the beginning of a breakdown of the old impersonality of technological medicine.

Many Christians believe that the New Age, with its welcome of exotic spiritualities and self-improvement techniques, is a full-blown conspiracy to subvert both the Christian faith and also the whole of Western society. Siegel is seen as using Eastern meditative techniques and their possible connections with yoga and Hinduism, while Krieger is supposed to be subverting people with occult methods which are, by definition, in league with the devil. Nothing in the books by either author, however, makes this *feel* true in any sense. Their motivations may not be Christian in a full sense, but each is promoting something good which Christians can surely work with.

No doubt there are many aspects of the New Age movement which are either misguided or plain silly—or possibly evil. But the impression I have gained from reading many books on the New Age movement is that there is no conspiracy—only a pot-pourri of ideas, beliefs and ideas for changing the world and which range from the dangerous to the helpful. Siegel and Krieger belong to the helpful end of the spectrum, even though not everyone would agree with everything they say.

Spiritual experience and the New Age

In continuing this reflection on the New Age and its importance for a new culture of healing within society, the reader should consider two areas of direct spiritual experience which are relevant to healing and which are frequently discussed in New Age literature. These are not experiences which the movement can in any sense own, but they are spontaneous spiritual experiences, for which the New Age movement offers one inter-pretative framework.

The first of these spontaneous religious experiences is associated with severe illness and near-death; the second is centred around an encounter with or a sense of guidance by entities who are felt to be assisting the individual through life. It would be convenient and more comfortable to ignore these and other spiritual experiences on the grounds that from the Christian point of view they occur to people who have no denominational faith and are thus sometimes outside the orbit of orthodox religious life. Many Christian writers do, in fact, ignore the religious experience of non-Christians as if it were of no importance. But the impact of these experiences on the culture of healing in society is of considerable interest and importance.

In any gathering of people today, there is a good chance that at least one individual will have had or know someone who has had a 'near-death experience'. The details of such experiences need not detain us here and the interested reader may be referred to the vast literature devoted to this subject[4]. In brief, individuals at the point of death are led down a long tunnel to a place of light where they are welcomed by loved ones who have already died. A Christ-figure helps them to see the course of their life and understand it in a new way. The common message of all the people who have encountered this experience is that the place of light was so beatific that they had no wish to return and that 'coming back' was hard and painful.

Christian commentaries on such experiences do exist, but for the most part the task of interpretation has fallen to people who write from the New Age perspective. Their reflections on these experiences tend to introduce ideas of *karma*—the working out of a previous life—and reincarnation, which have little place in a Christian framework of understanding. But the experiences themselves are greater than any of the interpretations given. Indeed for most people words are simply inadequate to describe what they have known. On waking, they claim to be no longer afraid of death, and indeed their lives and attitudes are changed by this encounter.

Other experiences encountered at the time of severe illness and near-death are a little more mundane; 'floating on the ceiling' as nurses and doctors fight to save their lives on the trolley below is an experience reported by many people. But even this experience, with its implied separation of body and awareness, can help people as they try to come to terms with the materialistic ideas of Western scientific culture—a culture which suggests that consciousness is linked with brain function and that any kind of awareness away from the body is impossible.

The second area of raw spiritual experience which is increasingly common in Western culture is the sense of being in touch with and guided by an intelligence or intelligences beyond our own. Once again many people with such an experience will be led to interpret it in the light of New Age ideology. Equally Christian ways of understanding this do exist, however. For example, a strong sense of guidance is as much a feature of a 'born again' Christian as it is of many non-churchgoing people who have become attuned to someone or something beyond themselves guiding and leading them. The former will speak of the guidance of the Holy Spirit while the latter may use any number of interpretations according to choice. One acquaintance of mine immersed in a spiritualist culture speaks of 'those upstairs' and, as we have seen in our brief survey of Spiritualism, there are many people who claim to have spirit guides. Equally, many Christians who do not use the language of being guided 'by the Holy Spirit' will speak of a personal guardian angel helping them, or they may claim to be guided by God himself.

New Age beliefs have contributed to an awareness on the part of many people of feelings of spiritual guidance, but the experiences themselves are not therefore to be interpreted within New Age categories alone. Instead they form a part of the spiritual experience of considerable numbers of people in Western society, from many walks of life.

The implications of spiritual experience

The almost forcible encounter with a spiritual dimension through a near-death experience is, as we have indicated, both unsettling and life-changing. Many people do not reach the point of being able to articulate what has happened to them, let alone attach the experience to a religious system, New Age or Christian. Nevertheless, they are aware of a vast gulf between their new spiritual perceptions and those of the people around them.

The literature does indicate, however, that they bring into their personal lives many of the positive aspects of the experience. These include an awareness of an eternal spiritual dimension which has now become 'home', a freedom from the fear of death, and the importance of love in relationships. The loving encounter with departed relatives and friends as well as the 'Christ-figure', through whom a new perspective of their lives was obtained, changes their sense of what is important and what is trivial in life. Not infrequently, individuals from this point on devote themselves to a life of service which reflects something of that transcendent love and acceptance encountered in the experience. Some of these people may find their way into churches, but people who have had direct spiritual experiences are not always comfortably accommodated in the institutional church.

For many people, an encounter with a being or beings to guide them stays at the level of a feeling of reassurance. For the Christian, a direct experience which is interpreted to mean that God or Christ is with them on life's journey will lead to a greater confidence and trust that whatever happens they are never abandoned. Armed with this confidence they may feel free to love and care more, rather in the same way as the person who has glimpsed the reality of the life beyond. For a person who interprets a similar experience in line with New Age beliefs, there is also a new commitment to love and joy, but for different reasons.

The much quoted maxim that we create our own realities is a summary of the teaching of the spirit guides widely quoted in New Age literature. If we cultivate attitudes of joy, love and peace then that is the reality we will encounter around us. This principle will probably not do from a Christian point of view, as it takes no real account of the existence of evil and the need to face and overcome it in ourselves and others. But it is not without value. It has influenced the style of writing and teaching of Bernie Siegel, with his emphasis on the need to develop positive attitudes of love and self-affirmation while simultaneously defeating the negative effects of fear and hatred. There is, I believe, sufficient in that genre of writing with which Christians can identify to a large degree, even though they may stand aside from some of its conclusions.

New Age: an assessment

In this chapter I have looked at two manifestations of a New Age approach to healing. I have also touched on two areas of direct spiritual experience which are frequently referred to in New Age writing about matters of the spirit. In making this selection, however, a vast edifice of belief and practice which comes under the umbrella of New Age has been passed over without examination of any kind.

From a Christian perspective I have found plenty with which to disagree. There seems to be a failure to take the reality of evil seriously, there is an obsessive concern with the inner state of the individual, and a difficulty in dealing with weakness and failure. Enough has been said, however, to indicate there are at least some aspects of New Age culture that can receive a cautious welcome by a Christian believer. That some parts are less than satisfactory does not mean, I feel, that the whole edifice has to be cast aside.

Indeed, it would be wrong to suggest that the New Age is a single entity, since many of the activities labelled as 'New Age', such as alternative medicine, have their origins in places and times long before the movement could be said to have begun. If all New Age practices are considered together, then it is because they all form part of a protest against the mainstream ideas of so-called modern civilization.

One key element of New Age teaching is that each person creates his or her own reality by the attitudes he or she possesses. I have suggested that this is dangerous ; it ignores the mystery and tragedy of evil, and furthermore it tempts people into a *laisser-faire* approach to the problems of the world. It has to be acknowledged that New Age people have often shown far more concern for the world and the environment than many Christians, but the existence and problem of evil can easily be marginalized if you have in a comfortable, middle-class, Western lifestyle—though it comes very close if you are disadvantaged or poor and struggling to make ends meet.

Furthermore, a solution to the problem of evil which has long been part of Eastern religious systems, namely that human beings are working out the *karma* (the sum of experience) of previous lifetimes, does not seem a satisfactory answer to the problem, and that doctrine widely held among New Age believers, together with a belief in reincarnation, represents a gulf which is not easy for Christians or others within Western culture to cross.

Conclusion

Is there a bridge between the New Age movement and Christianity? The answer has to be that in health and healing, there certainly is potential. Much of the writing about adopting attitudes of love and joy towards the world and other people makes a lot of sense and can be heard by anyone. It is in areas where the New Age has little or nothing to say that problems arise. Christians must have reservations about the way that evil seems to be totally or partially ignored; Christian teaching has always emphasized the existence of evil, not particularly in the sense of demonic forces but in the deliberate choice of evil even when it works against the obvious benefit of an individual. And the defeat of evil is never a matter merely of adopting positive attitudes but rather of aligning ourselves with one who himself has fought evil through the Cross—Jesus Christ.

CHAPTER 9

Christian Healing–Origins and History

The distinctive style of healing that is called Christian looks back to the activity and beliefs of Jesus in the first century. In past generations, certain Christian commentators have found the heavy emphasis on the accounts of miracles in the Gospels something of an embarrassment, and they have sought various ways of explaining them away.

The writing of the German theologian, Rudolf Bultmann, in the 1930s followed the lines of Christian exist-entialism and had little room for the idea that the healings of Jesus might actually have happened. The early nineteenth-century hymn writer, John Marriott, also reflected the beliefs of his generation, deliberately excluding a physical dimension to Jesus' healing when he wrote, 'health to the sick in mind, sight to the inly blind'. Such scepticism, even in Christian circles, can be traced back to the eighteenth-century philosophy of Enlightenment; miracles became unfashionable and unacceptable when there was a growing confidence in the laws of nature to explain the workings of the universe in a consistent fashion.

Over the generations, New Testament scholars have swung back to an acceptance of the broad truth of the healing miracles. There is also a fresh understanding of the way in which the accounts of the healing miracles fit into a consistent and coherent picture of Jesus and the way he affected his contemporaries, friend and foe alike.

Many presentations of the ministry and teaching of Jesus note the centrality of the teaching of the 'kingdom of God' (of 'heaven', in Matthew's Gospel). The kingdom is another word for the rule of God, the manifestation of God moving towards his people to give them the blessings of his salvation. The kingdom is not present in any final sense. It requires a response, a desire to receive it and become part of it. In proclaiming the kingdom Jesus was himself inviting individuals to enter it and know its reality within their lives.

Those who came into contact with Jesus' teaching and personality were also brought into contact with the power, forgiveness, healing and love which were all aspects of the kingdom of God. Perhaps the most striking example of this proclamation of the kingdom and its impact on individuals is in the stories of Jesus eating and drinking with tax gatherers (collaborators with the hated Romans) and prostitutes. Our imagination has to fill in some of the detail but we can see in our minds Jesus gathering around him this marginalized group. There was ,by the very fact of eating with them, a proclamation that God's forgiveness was freely available and could be experienced at that moment. Such an offer of forgiveness would also have been backed up by a tangible sense of the nearness of God mediated through the words and presence of Jesus.

It is also clear that we are to understand healing as an aspect of the reality of the kingdom. When giving his disciples instructions to go out and proclaim the nearness of the kingdom, Jesus tells them simultaneously to 'heal the sick, raise the dead, cleanse those who have leprosy... (Matthew 10:7–8). Thus our understanding of the kingdom of God is of a reality not just talked about, but made tangibly and powerfully present by Jesus and his disciples in forgiveness and healing to those who opened themselves to it by faith. In short, the healing miracles were signs and pointers to the reality of God's kingdom breaking through into the world. Both healing and forgiveness were part of the reality of God's salvation which Jesus was announcing to the world.

Jesus' teaching possesses a great simplicity which in many ways is summed up in his words at the beginning of Mark's gospel, 'The Kingdom of God is near, repent and believe the good news.' The only qualification for receiving this kingdom is to turn around (the original sense of 'repentance') and to have a new attitude of faith, trust and repentance which can receive what is being offered by God. This new attitude includes letting go of all selfishness and self-centred sin, which is a mark of a person cut off from God. Once the kingdom, the movement of God towards each individual, becomes alive and active within the person who has received it, there is a corresponding revolution in that individual's attitudes and behaviour toward others.

The parables of the kingdom are word pictures of the new situation that arises during and after the kingdom is received. The person who goes and sells everything to buy the pearl of great price or the field with treasure in it is the one who has discovered what it is to receive the kingdom. The prodigal son experiences the kingdom as a reconciliation with God, after wasting everything on riotous living. The good soil that receives the seed of the kingdom brings forth abundant fruit. The whole thrust of Jesus' teaching about behaviour and ways of living can be interpreted as a working out of the implications of kingdom living. In short, to know God in Christ moving towards humanity changes everything; it releases in human beings the same love and forgiveness towards others that they have received from God.

The miracle stories in different ways reveal the power of God's kingdom at work in Jesus, healing disease and defeating the activity of spirits which cause disease. In contrast with these references to the power of Jesus to heal, it should be noted how little power he possessed for himself. His power was used to empower others. The model of greatness and power he leaves with his disciples is that of the slave, and this principle is vividly portrayed in his act of washing his disciples' feet. The crucifixion is also a dramatic demonstration of the principle of power in powerlessness, of love in total vulnerability.

The Book of Acts shows the very early church discovering that the healing work of Christ continued through his disciples. For Paul, the church as the 'body of Christ' possessed the Holy Spirit who distributed all the gifts, including healing, to individual members of the church. All the gifts, when exercised, were to build up and further the work of the church in the world. But already by the time the Letter of James was written, there were signs of a process which was to attach charismas or individual gifts to those who held positions of leadership. However well the healing ministry of the church survived through the centuries, it still became attached to structures of defined authority along with the administration of the sacraments (baptism, confirmation, communion, and so on). A sense that the work of Christ continued through every baptized member within the church soon became lost and is only now being rediscovered today.

Christian healing through the ages

Many Christians believe that Christian healing has only been recovered by the church in our own day. In fact there is a continuous thread which binds the healing miracles of the New Testament to the ministries of today. Much of the information about this ministry is, however, in the byways of church history. But it is helpful to look briefly at the way Christian healing has been expressed at different times in the past, since the variety of settings in which it is found provides a commentary on the situation today.

From the days of the early church until the end of the Middle Ages in about AD 1500, there was a focus on healing through the holiness of particular places and people. The ancient pagan world into which Christianity was born after its severance from its Jewish roots was a world full of places consecrated to particular gods and goddesses. Much pagan religious observance consisted of making pilgrimages to local sanctuaries. With the conversion of the Roman world in the fourth century, there was a need to provide similar places of religious focus, places of particular holiness.

Soon, encouragement was given to the setting up of holy places which commemorated the site of the tombs of particular martyrs, most of whom had died in the fifty years prior to the conversion of the emperor Constantine in AD313. These tombs, the places which contained the relics of saints, were sites of great holiness to pilgrims. Somehow, through the presence of these relics, they believed that they were in a place where heaven became especially close to the earth. Coming to such a place at times of illness was a natural step to take and miracles were recorded all over the Christian world at these tombs. Augustine of Hippo, who was not particularly interested in healing at the start of his Christian life, records the amazing miracles that took place in his diocese when a relic of the martyr, Stephen, was brought to his own town of Hippo in North Africa in 424. People in the West were later than those in the eastern part of the empire to experience healing at martyrs' tombs. Once established, however, this mode of healing survived in the Western church right up to the end of the Middle Ages.

The tradition of the holy man who prayed for the sick was also found in the Christian East from the earliest times. The holy man is associated with the monastic tradition which began in the fourth century in Egypt and spread from there to all parts of the Christian world. In Syria in the sixth century the local holy man was normally a hermit who lived apart from the rest of society. By doing so, he would act as an independent agent, mediating the unseen heavenly realms to the local communities by giving counsel and praying for the sick. He would also plead on their behalf to the secular authorities who respected his role in society. The writings of Pope Gregory the Great, who wrote at the end of the sixth century, are a rich source of stories of healings which took place at the hands of individuals before and during his lifetime. It is striking how few of the miracles recorded are ascribed to laymen, though some do exist, and none at all were accomplished by women.

The Venerable Bede writing in England in the eighth century also told many stories of religious heroes who effected healings through the laying on of hands, especially Cuthbert of Durham. One mediaeval figure who possessed a gift of healing was Bernard of Clairvaux, who went on a preaching tour through Germany in 1146–47, effecting many miracles.

Generally speaking, though, the high Middle Ages saw the focus of healing return to the religious shrines, where no living person was involved. The pilgrimage centres of Britain, Canterbury, Hereford, Lincoln and other places, have left numerous accounts of individuals who travelled along the muddy roads to receive healing as they prayed at the shrines of the saints buried and commemorated in those centres. Transformations, both mental and physical, seem to have occurred at these holy places. A dynamic form of healing was alive and well in the mediaeval Christian shrines of England.

From the Reformation until modern times

In the early sixteenth century, the destruction by Henry VIII of the old medieval shrines and centres of pilgrimage brought to an end a style of healing focused on holy relics. In fact, the age of miracle-working shrines had severely declined in importance from its heyday in thirteenth-century Britain. Perhaps Henry was merely giving the *coup de grâce* to a system of Christian healing that had begun to die two centuries earlier. The way was left open for the rediscovery of the style of Christian healing where the personal gifts of individuals came to the fore.

Outside the control of the church were numerous 'wise men' or 'sorcerers' who, according to Robert Burton writing in 1621, were to be found in every village. One remarkable figure who appeared briefly in England in 1666 was Walter Greatrakes. Born in Ireland, Greatrakes was championed in Britain by the intellectuals and scientists of the day, including Robert Boyle and other members of the Royal Society. Although a Christian, who believed the power he possessed came from God, he made no attempt to operate under the supervision of the church of his day. Even more important for the history of Christian healing was George Fox (1624–91), whose lost *Book of Miracles* survived only in summary form; even so, it left a mine of healing stories which deserve to be better known.

The eighteenth century represents a low point in the history of Christian healing, with the forces of rationalism everywhere in the ascendant. John Wesley, although otherwise counteracting these trends through his passionate preaching, does not seem himself to have practised a healing ministry. His *Journal* records a series of astonishing phenomena among his congregations, paralleled by the contemporary 'Toronto Blessing', but these were evidences of conversion and conviction of sin. There is, however, evidence that the first generation of Methodist believers prayed for the sick.

The nineteenth-century healing scene was dominated by the emergence of Lourdes in southern France as a pilgrimage centre for healing miracles. This emergence marks the rediscovery of the holy place as a focus of healing where no human agents are involved. Lourdes has a unique place in any presentation of Christian healing, and the certified miracles, though not numerous, should be studied by anyone who doubts the extraordinary power of faith. Further-more, one suspects that for every miracle recognized by the International Medical Bureau, with its rigorous medical checks and examinations, there are also many hundreds if not thousands of people who experience considerable help and healing.

But however significant the Christian healing in Lourdes has been, both in the nineteenth century and today, there seems to be a clinging on to a style of healing which reaches back to the Middle Ages. Some people must inevitably come back from a pilgrimage with their condition completely unchanged and no one knows how many of them might be helped by other methods or styles of Christian healing on offer today. (We shall be looking at some of these in the next chapter.) In short, the focus on Lourdes to the exclusion of other centres of healing is not particularly helpful to the sick, who may need to explore the immense variety of the healing styles within the Church and through which Christ is seen to heal today.

Exercising an individual gift of healing was by no means extinct in the nineteenth century, and one person in particular may be mentioned to represent this kind of care. He was the maverick priest-monk, Father Ignatius (1837–1908), who sought to revive the Benedictine Order and who spent most of his ministry as a missionary deacon. Several stories of healings are told about him. One account in his biography tells of the illness of a Mrs Mar, who was on the edge of death from 'consumption of the stomach'. Father Ignatius spent a few minutes with her and then, after she had given assent to her belief in Jesus Christ, commanded her to arise. She recovered immediately and he left the family with the instructions that they were to send out for a beefsteak for the patient that evening and that Mrs Mar was to appear at the early celebration at St Bartholomew's, the neighbouring church, with her family the following morning. The attending doctor, it is recorded, was so shocked that he took to his bed for six weeks with a nervous complaint!

The twentieth-century revival of healing

The revival of the Christian healing ministry in our present century seems to have two main streams. In the first, a group of individuals, some of them extraordinarily gifted healers in their own right, founded institutions in the first twenty years of this century which were devoted to the cause of Christian healing. In the second stream, the Pentecostal churches, which began to be effective in this country around 1910, started a distinctive, exuberant style of healing which eventually in the 1960s flowed into all the mainstream churches as the charismatic movement.

The twentieth-century revival in its institutional form is associated with such figures as James Moore Hickson and Dorothy Kerrin. Both these pioneering figures had a distinctive personal ministry which, in Hickson's case, was world-wide. In 1905, he founded 'The Society of Emmanuel', later to become 'The Divine Healing Mission' in 1933. Dorothy Kerrin's ministry began in 1912 with the remarkable case of her own healing at the point of death from a tubercular disease. She received at the same time a personal call to the healing ministry. She went on to found the important healing centre of Burrswood and presided over it until her death in 1963. Both these pioneers were careful to be obedient to the church and seek the blessing of its authorities at every point of their subsequent ministry.

Other organizations of this century have been the Guild of Health, founded in 1904 by Percy Dearmer and Conrad Noel, and the Guild of St Raphael, founded in 1915. All these organizations, together with the many healing homes which have subsequently emerged, have preserved their own distinct ethos according to the vision of their founders and the style that developed with the subsequent leadership. Their independence has been both a strength and a weakness. On the one hand they have continued to witness to the reality of Christian healing, regardless of the thinking of the wider church. On the other, their independence has meant that the health of the organizations has depended, perhaps too heavily, on the personalities in charge. When the history of the healing movement in this country is fully written up it will no doubt focus largely on the personalities involved, both in their strengths and in their weaknesses.

The advent of the charismatic movement from the mid-1960s helped to breathe life not only into the churches but also into the somewhat flagging healing movement. The style of this movement owed much to the older Pentecostal churches which had been practising healing along with other spiritual gifts since the years just before the First World War.

These Pentecostal churches maintained a considerable profile in their early years, partly as a result of the Welsh Revival of 1904 and partly following the American Pentecostal explosion of 1906. Thanks to the crusades of the Welsh Jeffreys brothers from 1925–35, crusade evangelism and public healing was kept in public awareness. The style of conversion was forceful and the worship exuberant, and these crusades reached many who were untouched by the more intellectual churches. Many Caribbean immigrants in the 1940s and 1950s found their way into membership of these churches, finding the older churches stuffy and off-putting. But Pentecostalism as a whole became less visible after the period of the Jeffreys' crusades, and their strict, fundamentalist, exclusive position meant that their distinctive theology made little impact on the rest of the churches in Britain.

In contrast the charismatic movement has learnt to co-exist with the hierarchical structure of the mainstream denominations, including Roman Catholicism. Although it might be claimed that the charismatic movement has recently shifted back to a more fundamentalist stance, the overall energy it has given to the whole church, including its healing activities, has been positive and life-enhancing.

The contemporary scene

To bring this brief history of the Christian healing movement to a close, it can be said that, in Britain at any rate, Christian healing possesses a vitality greater than ever before in its history. Every diocese of the Church of England has a healing adviser and parishes are constantly encouraged to explore the implications of prayer and ministry to the sick. Many healing organizations and homes of healing enjoy wide support, and magazines and books flow from the presses. The situation is not, however, without some serious difficulties, and it is important to address these briefly.

The first problem that the Christian healing scene finds is that it is a victim of its own success. In seeking to provide a response to the demand for healing of all kinds, some churches have become identified with manifestations of Christian healing which are crude, manipulative and money-seeking. It is not difficult for a thinking Christian to find a reason for pushing aside the whole phenomenon on the grounds that some expressions of this ministry are banal, anti-intellectual or even frightening. Some of the grounds for this complaint will be further explored in the next chapter.

The second problem is that the whole Christian academic tradition in universities and theological colleges seems to have effectively boycotted the subject of healing, as being unworthy of serious study. Those people gifted in healing who are also involved in church ministry are unable to provide the intellectual underpinning for their work which would allow them to communicate with thoughtful theologians and members of the medical profession. Although there are some doctors interested and concerned in the Christian healing ministry, there is no literature available which is able to bridge the considerable cultural divide between medicine and Christian ministry.

Conclusion

I end this chapter reviewing the history of Christian healing on a somewhat negative note as a way of indicating the considerable task that stills awaits Christian healing as it moves into the next century. As a distinctive, powerful expression of the gospel of Jesus Christ at work in the church and the world today, it has yet to conquer the heart and mind of the wider church. Until that victory is won, it will remain on the fringes of the church's life, however many people are blessed and healed through its care.

CHAPTER 10

The Cultures of Christian Healing

In a study on the Christian healing movement which I wrote some nine years ago[25], I found myself compelled to question the traditional way that commentators characterize the Christian healing ministry. There was a tendency to see the movement as possessing two main strands, charismatic and sacramental.

I queried this division because it presented two concepts which were not strictly comparable. The word 'charismatic' describes a type of spirituality; 'sacramental', however, is descriptive of the setting in which prayer an healing take place, one that is open to divine grace through special rites and ceremonies. It is not in itself a type of spirituality.

I would make the claim that a more precise way of distinguishing between the varieties of healing ministry would be to look at the spiritual activities of those who practice them. The healing movement could therefore be described as a spectrum with two main strands. The first of these leans towards an extrovert, charismatic style of spirituality and the other towards a meditational style, where silence and stillness are valued.

At each end of the spectrum there were some in my research whose claim to possess a Christian ministry of healing was questionable. In the case of extreme charismatics there were examples of individuals whose awareness of being part of a wider church body was almost non-existent. Their individual style was so personalized and independent that it had become corrupted by its failure to allow any kind of criticism or self-scrutiny. It is among such practitioners that there are still some people who refuse to allow co-operation with doctors and who will counter all criticism as being 'Satan-inspired'. The extreme examples I found at the other end of the spectrum were those who merged into spiritualist or New Age practices and who seemed to be using the title 'Christian' as a label of convenience.

The task today of drawing precise boundaries is not easy, and indeed there are those who occupy a grey area where the claim of being Christian at all is not easy to verify. However, the position of this book is to give groups and individuals the benefit of the doubt, rather than exclude them because some people find their theology or practices uncongenial.

Charismatic healing

In the last chapter we looked briefly at the history this century of the Pentecostal and charismatic movements. Although I have criticized some practitioners of this style of spirituality and healing practice on theological and practical grounds, it is in fact hard to imagine how Christian healing as a whole would have achieved its prominence in this last decade of the twentieth century without the important contribution of the charismatic style of spirituality. Certainly I cannot imagine this book having been written had not my interest in Christian healing been aroused in large part by those involved in Pentecostal and charismatic styles of healing.

My previous book[25] describes how it was in a Pentecostal setting that my wife found a partial but nevertheless significant relief from her rheumatoid arthritis. Since that time we have been in touch with the charismatic style of spirituality, at the same time being aware of the wider dimension of the Christian healing movement.

The charismatic style of spirituality is rooted in the Pentecostal churches, as already described. The charismatic movement began its life in this country in the mid- to late-1960s, when the distinctive experiences hitherto known only to Pentecostalism began to be manifest in mainstream churches. The most notable characteristic of this spirituality is the gift of 'speaking in tongues', (speaking in unknown languages) which is believed to be a replication of the gift to the apostles on the day of Pentecost, ten days after Christ was taken to heaven. Alongside this gift, the charismatic movement has become aware of a variety of other biblical gifts such as prophecy, discernment and healing.

According to the Jungian map of the psyche expounded by the American Christian writer, Morton Kelsey, the Holy Spirit 'covers and fills the psyche, bringing harmony out of the tension of discordant contents and spirits, integrating much of the unconsciousness that often appears as evil darkness.... ' In short, the charismatic experience is itself healing, in the sense that it is a participation in a new spiritual wholeness and harmony.

A further definition of the charismatic experience is offered by Martin Israel, a well-known writer on spiritual themes. He speaks of the experience as 'an opening of the personality to the warmth of a universal relationship, so that a person who was previously shut in himself, emotionally inhibited and unable to pray with real conviction because of stultifying agnosticism or personal pride, is now released to show himself to the world, even as a child'. He describes it further as 'a dynamic response to God's love'. Simultaneously, the experience has the capacity to awaken gifts and abilities that in other contexts would be understood as psychic gifts, but in the context of the individual's relationship with the Holy Spirit are seen to be spiritual and God-centred.

The charismatic experience of conversion is described most typically as the baptism of the Holy Spirit. With it comes a new freedom in prayer and worship together with a tremendous sense of joy. The most notable feature of charismatic spirituality is a completely new sense of corporate prayer, accompanied by music and singing. The movement has produced its own distinctive cultural identity in its music. It is said that as much as one third of all Anglican Christians are caught up in the movement to some extent, and the churches that are its centres, such as Holy Trinity, Brompton in London, are places of incredible growth as well as of sacrificial commitment and giving.

Within the context of charismatic worship there is frequently prayer offered for the sick. That healings occur, I have no doubt. To describe the mechanism involved means recalling some of the findings in earlier chapters. Large groups have always been susceptible to heightened suggestibility, and if an illness is in any way caused by destructive attitudes then the sense of spiritual and group energy flowing through the meeting may well be able to shift the 'block' at a deep level and promote the process of healing.

The same spiritual energy may also, in certain situations, activate deep self-healing mechanisms within the individual which will turn the course of the illness. The charismatic literature reports even that legs can lengthened after prayer. While I have never witnessed such a manifestation, what I have witnessed tells me that it would be foolish to limit what the mind activated by prayer can achieve in healing the body. The mechanism of self-healing through the mind is well documented, and I believe that healing offered through prayer uses this mechanism, although with a complexity and depth that our models of understanding can do little to grasp.

For many people, charismatic healing in a large meeting fulfils an important need for physical and emotional healing. It can, however, be a somewhat blunt instrument, and many individuals may not be helped since their illnesses and underlying needs require more individual attention.

As a next step, prayer-counselling may be offered to an individual, normally by two people. From the point of view of charismatic theology, the main gift to be evoked here is that of discernment. The counsellors will pray to be given insight into the root problem of the individual before them. They will then bring the resources and power of prayer to break such problems as a dependency on the past or some grief that has never been healed. When the gift of discernment is exercised, an individual can be released in a comparatively short period, particularly when the person seeking to be helped actively accepts the paradigm or framework of interpretation of the counsellors.

So far this portrait of charismatic healing has been enthusiastic and positive, but there is another side. The positive health-giving aspects of charismatic healing are very easily distorted and turned upside down, whether in a large crowd setting or in a counselling group. The same suggestibility that makes healing a possibility for an individual in a large crowd can also be the means of exploitation and coercion. When vast healing crusades are organized, a lot of money is needed, and the only place that money can come from is the individuals who attend them. Quite apart from seeking to take money from vulnerable people, the leaders of healing crusades can all too easily reduce the 'healing' to a crude, manipulative technique which leaves the sick that remain sick feeling devastated and burdened with guilt because they have not become well.

When healing methods become a matter of using the right technique, regardless of the sensitivities and needs of the individual members of the congregation, we come back to an old theme—the misuse of power. To stand up in front of thousands of people, who believe, rightly or wrongly, that you are a 'healer' and able to affect them at a very sensitive point in their lives, is a very intoxicating experience. But the spiritual dangers are immense, and burn-out must be a constant problem. Although the focus is supposed to be on God who does the healing, the temptation is always going to be to use the crowd dynamic in a crude way to create an atmosphere of power with little or no spiritual content. In other words, instead of being opened up to the activity of the Spirit of God by the prayer and sensitive guidance of the crowd by the leader, there may be an experience of crowd power and energy which feeds the leader's ego.

A major requirement in such meetings, therefore, is humility— humility which will constantly remind the leader and the group that a genuine encounter with the Spirit of God can only be achieved when there has been a costly surrender of pride, love of power and self-importance. The comment about Jesus being someone who used power in the context of his own powerlessness should be recalled.

Similar but less obvious temptation exists for the charismatic counsellor who is dealing with an individual. The use of two people in a counselling situation is a check in the exercise of the gift of discernment. Discernment can be a genuine short-cut into the heart of an individual's problem, but once again it can also be the exercise of human power, with the authority of the Holy Spirit used to support it. The charismatic culture becomes dangerous when anyone is allowed to claim direct access to infallible truth or the will of God without fear of contradiction. To quote Martin Israel again, the potentially negative side of charismatic spirituality tends to 'brush aside, if not totally ignore, any other approach to truth'. Because the emotional and intuitive sides of the personality have come to the fore, reason is put on one side and 'other aspects of truth... are then either ignored or else assailed as the work of dark, demonic forces that govern the material world'.

Healing through meditative prayer

The charismatic culture is a powerful and important mechanism through which many people have found the way to a spiritual power of healing. An even older tradition of spirituality known to the church is that of meditation. It is a spiritual discipline that seeks the same reordering of the psyche that the charismatics look for and that will align our spirits to the Spirit of God. But, unlike the charismatic style, meditation thrives on silence and stillness. Also, although meditation groups exist, much of the work of meditation is accomplished by individuals on their own.

As would be expected, there is more than one method of Christian meditation. One classic Christian tradition was formulated by Ignatius, a sixteenth-century writer and mystic who both founded the Society of Jesus (the Jesuits) and began a system of prayer which still bears his name. It consisted of using the active imagination as a way of entering the events of the Gospel story and allowing the life and spirit of Jesus to enter the mind and heart.

Eastern Orthodox methods of prayer centre on the Jesus prayer, the repetition of the prayer 'Lord Jesus Christ, Son of God, have mercy upon me, a sinner'. This prayer aids mediation like a kind of mantra and, by stilling the heart and mind, it helps the one praying to be opened to the spirit of Christ.

Other methods take techniques from Eastern religions— concentrating on breathing, for instance—in an attempt to find a new awareness of the workings of the unconscious mind. All these methods of meditation and stillness attempt to make the individual who seeks to be a vehicle of God's healing power more effective in this ministry.

Of all the written accounts of healing ministries, and there are many, the one that describes most movingly the spiritual preparation required to exercise it is that given by J. Cameron Peddie, a Scottish Presbyterian minister who began his influential activities in the late 1940s. He reasoned that if God were to use him for a healing ministry then he needed to prepare himself by offering the whole of his personality to God—body, mind and spirit. His preparation consisted of an hour a day from eleven till midnight keeping a 'Watch with Christ'. He would name every physical feature of his body, all the different aspects of his mind, and the depths of his spirit to God, so that they could be recreated by God and used in his service. This preparation lasted for five years until Peddie became convinced that he was ready to begin what was then a pioneering healing ministry in Scotland. His work, made more difficult by the fact that no one initially understood or shared his particular calling, shows that giftedness in healing needs to be backed by dedication and consecration to God, so that pride and power-seeking cannot be allowed to interfere with it.

Sacramental healing

The word 'sacrament' is used by Christians to refer to special symbolic actions, believed to be God-given, which show God's presence in the world. The two most common sacraments are baptism and holy communion. In the older churches—Anglican, Roman Catholic and Orthodox—the word is extended to include five other rituals performed by a priest, one of which is the anointing of a sick person on the forehead with a specially blessed oil. Sacramental anointing is believed to be a channel for God's power; there is also an expectation that the prayer and faith of the sick person will help in making God's healing power effective.

There will usually, in practice, be other praying people involved, both ordained and lay. Sacramental healing also naturally links the sick person with the whole praying church, past and present. This sense of belonging to God's praying and timeless church can be powerfully effective for many sick people.

The sacramental style of healing is most appropriate for Christians who are practising members of the church. Even here it is necessary to make some qualification. For example, has the sick person been immersed in the culture of the sacraments over a long period of time? The parish communion 'culture', with its emphasis on the corporate body of Christ within the community, can sometimes diminish the power of the sacramental elements of bread and wine. Conversely, congregations with a strong sacramental life may lack the corporate dimension which is so important in providing the right supporting environment for an effective healing ministry.to individuals; they have often learnt to focus on the role of the priest in the proceedings., under the influence of a centuries-old theology which sees priests exalted above the congregation they serve. Thus an effective theology of sacramental healing will need to find a balance between affirming the power of God in the sacramental action and preserving the vibrant sense of the healing 'body of Christ' at work in the Christian congregation.

Sacramental healing nevertheless remains a crucially important aspect of the healing ministry, particularly when the distortions mentioned above are not present. Through it, a link is established with Christians all through the ages back to the earliest times of the church. Priests do not anoint to exercise a particular gift of their own. Rather, in the sacrament they are joining together the prayers of the church with their own prayers, and mediating the promised grace of God to sick people. As with any sacrament, there is an 'objectivity' about the action, a sense that God can use it in ways that go beyond the understanding. The decline of sacramental anointing as a sacrament of healing is a cause for regret. A renewal of its understanding and its use in settings which have already been carefully prepared to be places of healing would be a great benefit and blessing to the church.

Conclusion

Healing ministries within a Christian context will vary from place to place. What has been offered in this chapter is a way to understand the various types of ministries that are encountered. I have spoken about healing ministries in terms of the spirituality within which healing takes place. I have also expressed my belief that Christian healing needs the involvement of many people,, either directly, or indirectly in prayer support to the healer.

Ultimately, the ministry of healing belongs to God. The more the action is taken away from an individual, who may get things wrong, the healthier it will be. In the last chapter we saw how Christ possessed the power to heal, but he himself was powerless to protect himself. The more the power to heal is shared by the church 'body' or group, the less danger there is of any individual becoming powerful and failing to see that he or she is only given power with which to empower others.

Also in this chapter I have spoken about the extremes that can occur in the healing ministry. These are dangerous and, where extreme positions are emphasized, unhelpful and even damaging distortions are likely to arise. Wholeness and balance are the key to effective healing, where an equilibrium is preserved between the personal and the impersonal, the corporate and the individual; and above all where the power of God can reach suffering people without that power being distorted by our own needs and inadequacies.

CHAPTER 11

The Christian Healing
Ministry in Practice

In this chapter I do not seek to provide success stories of healings I have known or read about. There are many books that do just that (although they may leave many questions unanswered) and, unfortunately, a list of success stories often gives a false impression. Few people, Christian or not, are wonderfully and painlessly healed in mind and body the instant they fall ill. Some may not recover from physical illness at all. What I want to do here is to concentrate on introducing the reader to the atmosphere and ethos of Christian ministry, and I intend to explore some of the issues that are involved in both receiving and giving a Christian healing ministry.

In doing this, distinctions will perhaps become clearer between this and the other healing styles encountered in this book. Christian healing, like all the healing examined so far, has its own particular culture, experience and language to describe reality. I hope that the reader without any background in this tradition will be able to penetrate the language and thought-forms of this culture, to understand the way that many contemporary Christians encounter this reality of healing power.

In the discussion about the ministry of Jesus, the point has been made that healing was always seen in the wider context of the 'kingdom'. Christian healing today will always stress that prayer is made not only for physical cure but also for a renewed vision and encounter with God. In their thinking, some Christians tend to

125

separate out words like forgiveness, salvation and healing, and yet there is a real sense in which these concepts all are part of a single reality—the kingdom of God.

In looking for healing, Christians are required to be open to the possibility that God may have other plans for them than the relief of symptoms. Their constant prayer to God in every situation, regardless of whether illness is present, is that his will may be done for them, in them and through them for the good of others. Such a prayer, if it is offered with sincerity, requires a readiness to do something about all the things that interfere with a person's relationship with God and others.

First, however, we need to look at the ways in which Christian healing is offered, and the changes that are sought in the individual who longs to receive it. Many problems arise when Christian healing is offered as a simple 'quick fix' to painful or distressing symptoms. If that is what is promised and it fails to occur, the one prayed for is left with a sense of betrayal and anger towards God. If on the other hand the prayer that is offered seeks the will of God in the individual's life, then that may become the most important concern. Through a changed perception of God's will, there will be a possibility of seeing an illness in a completely different way.

Preparing ourselves to receive healing

In Chapters 2 and 8, we saw how, even in a totally secular context, the way we regard illness makes a crucial difference in our ability to fight it. It will be no surprise then if, in a Christian context, people are encouraged to develop distinctive attitudes which are helpful, and banish those which are destructive or negative.

In the first place a Christian minister will urge upon an individual the need to look at his or her relationships, both present and past. The effect of broken relationships, especially when they lead to continuing bitterness, can be harmful. We do not just 'forgive those who trespass against us' because it is the right thing to do; we do it because we ourselves are harmed if we don't.

So often, an important area to be addressed is the relationship with parents. Few parents avoid hurting their children in some way, even if only a few actually abuse them physically or emotionally. The deep sense of grief for a lost or damaged childhood is not assuaged easily and patient counselling is needed. Talking through the events of the long-distant past is helpful, particularly as the talking gives people a new relationship with that past.

For example, a woman might be locked into a particular anger with her father, but the anger may be simply an evocation or memory of her feelings as a misunderstood teenager. What is important is to change her perception from the seventeen-year-old's attitude to that of the thirty-five-year-old mother she has become. She needs permission to feel angry at the weakness of her father or the crass insensitivity he showed, as well as to remember the pain of the incidents in question. Then, having relived the indignation of a teenager towards the event, she can turn her more mature outlook on to that time and understand it and the personalities involved.

From grief and anger there now comes compassion and understanding, with the new possibility of forgiveness. A Christian counsellor, especially when dealing with a person of active faith, may well then lead her into remembering the past once more in the context of prayer. The woman will be encouraged to relive the event and see Christ present. His response to the situation will be imagined and his forgiveness and compassion for all the participants involved will be sought. Such an evocation of the presence of Christ in a past incident helps the one seeking healing to break out of fixed and often stubborn attitudes towards the past. Power is given to allow the individual to move on, free of the damaging effects of the past.

If forgiveness of others is an important part of coming to terms with the past, another aspect is allowing ourselves to be forgiven. One does not invite people to seek forgiveness because it is a proven part of their healing but because it will always be part of Christian ministry to do so. A particularly striking case from my own experience some years ago concerns a woman who was starting to be afflicted with rheumatoid arthritis. She had two small children and was very frightened of the illness. My wife Frances and I were invited to see her and we talked at length about her background, her marriage and her faith. At the end of the first session she mentioned that at the age of eighteen she had had an abortion from a pregnancy by her boyfriend, who had now become her husband. She appeared to be calm about it, believing that she had let it go. The next time we saw her it was obvious that the abortion had not been let go, because it was the first thing she mentioned.

Frances then shared with her a picture that she had been given when we prayed on the previous occasion. She had seen Jesus holding this child in his arms. The woman gazed for a moment, a little nonplussed, and then said with a broken voice before bursting into tears, 'What a beautiful picture.' The picture given through prayer was an invitation to the woman to enter into a completely new relationship with the past. It was to be one which accepted the fact that a human life had been involved in the abortion. Thus forgiveness was needed for the situation, and the picture showed it was offered. In a way that we can only speculate about, both the tears and the prayer which followed this new realization effected complete physical healing of the arthritis.

In another more recent incident, the relationship that needed to be forgiven and restored involved myself as a parish priest. An older woman in the parish became ill. For some time there had been a problem in our relationship, a problem caused by the fact that everything I said to her seemed to be the wrong thing. Once a fear was established that I was going to say something to which she might take exception, things got steadily worse and more tense. Visiting her in her home I was once more faced with my own fears about our relationship. After a few safe opening remarks I offered to pray with her. During the prayer I was very conscious how my relationship with the woman was being healed. We were together in a place of prayer and love and that dissolved all the tension of our relationship. That healing of our relationship was itself a miracle, but after the event she also claimed that physical healing had begun at that moment. Clearly in both stories we can see how important it is both to forgive and be forgiven in the search for healing.

A further dimension to the search for Christian healing is the cultivation of the attitude called faith. It is a word much misunderstood, not least among committed Christians. The Greek word for faith, pistis, is one that carries the idea of confidence in the trustworthiness of the person who inspires such faith. There is little in the word to connect it with any idea of intellectual belief. The individual is called upon to be open, to be confident in the reliability of God, in short to be expectant. The fact that people use the word in the context of a wrestling with intellectual doubts is an indication that the Christian faith has become for many people a very over-intellectualized affair. The invitation by Jesus described in Chapter 9 was a call to trust and to be open to the activity of God. A similar call to have expectancy is a prerequisite to a prayer for healing. While healing may be the most obvious need of the individual, he or she is called upon to recognize that God is needed for all his gifts, including his forgiveness and love.

As already noted, it is when faith is understood in this wider sense that prayer will indeed release healing at some level. This is particularly true if we have allowed a scrutiny of ourselves to take place, letting go of those things—resentments, bitterness and fears—that affect and harm us. The experience of being prayed for by another Christian, whether on an individual basis or in a group, is a very powerful event. Even if only a little physical healing takes place, most will experience a new sense of purpose and direction, and a feeling that life is under God's control. With that, our relationship with our illness or disability can be changed and a new way of going forward may be found.

Critics of Christian healing prayer have suggested that any idea that death is 'the ultimate healer' is a refusal to admit failure. How can death be in any sense healing? Those who make this criticism fail to understand the many levels at which Christian healing is understood. Granted that physical healing is the most obvious goal, there may also be a new sense of the power and purpose of God at work in the life of an individual. The period immediately before death may resonate with a tremendous sense of joy, as unfinished business is completed, and there is a sense of expectation of moving to a new stage in one's relationship with God.

Death remains the great taboo in society, and healing which enables an individual to face it without fear is a healing indeed. Those who are involved in Christian healing need to hold on to an understanding of healing that can see God's will at work in pain, in Christ's experience of suffering and in the crucifixion itself. God's purposes were accomplished in all these events in the life of Jesus, and the faith of a Christian must be open and able to see that healing is not necessarily absent when physical healing does not take place. For many people there is an obvious paradox in the statement that death is the ultimate healing; this will always remain a paradox if they cannot come to see the glory of God in the one who predicted that, through his death, 'I will draw all men to myself'.

Mediating the healing of Christ

In this section, I want to move on from a consideration of the attitudes of one who comes for Christian healing to think about the way that all Christians can share in the healing process. I have always felt that the right to pray with another Christian belongs to clergy and lay people alike. The fact that a biblical passage, in Chapter 5 of the Letter of James, speaks of the 'elders' being called on to pray for the sick does not in any way change my feeling on this matter. The church to which James belonged was one where members were called on to 'confess their sins to each other and pray for each other so that you may be healed'. Thus there was formal and informal prayer for the sick, and both appeared effective.

Prayer in groups and in people's homes among ordinary Christians is as much a part of Christian ministry as formal healing services. The remarks that I make now about healing prayer for others is meant to apply as much to 'elders', those with a formal ministry, as to those ordinary Christians called to pray with others who are in some kind of need.

The first thing to be said has already been touched on in the previous chapter, namely that healing prayer is never something done alone. An individual may physically be alone with another person when prayer is made, but he or she needs to be part of a network of people who are praying for them and with them.

There are various reasons for this. The first is that for a Christian the insight that healing is given to the whole church is an important one as 'we are members one of another'. Prayer is also a protection from whatever evil may be in-volved in another person's suffering. This is a complex and difficult area, but in the intimate and close relationship that healing prayer can involve, we can become 'oppressed' in various ways with 'psychic debris'. Thus we need some spiritual armour provided by our own preparation and that of our prayer supporters. Thirdly and more importantly, people need the protection of prayer to prevent them ever becoming convinced that the ministry is somehow their own and not that of Jesus and his church, of which they are representatives.

It is a regrettable fact that ministries do go astray when individuals claim power for themselves. There are some recorded cases of ministries where individuals, finding themselves at the centre of an apparently powerful healing ministry, begins to show signs of mental instability and theological extremism, simply because they see themselves as subordinate to no one and certainly not subject to any checking by co-workers. The power which may have begun as divine power ends as human power, corrupting the holder in the process.

The second aspect of ministry within a Christian group is the quality of the relationship with the one who comes for healing prayer. Although Christians can be influenced by secular models of counselling, I believe they have a different model to guide them. There is a characteristic of 'spiritual intimacy', which marks the quality of the relationship between the minister and the one who comes for ministry. This expression describes the aspect of prayer that undergirds the relationship and which releases it to have a greater degree of closeness than the secular models might feel appropriate or desirable. I certainly believe that the relationship of prayer between Christians can bring them into a closer intimacy than anything else. In this closeness there is an understanding of the meaning of love in a Christian context, a love that is to do with showing the love of God for an individual.

This is also a love that genuinely seeks the highest and the best for the other and never tries to possess or manipulate. Many people come for ministry who have never known what it is to be totally accepted in love by another person. Love is itself a powerful healer in whatever context it is found. Churches should provide far more in the way of love as a preparation and follow-up for the intimacy of healing prayer. But in this talk about love, wisdom is needed. An offer of love or 'intimacy' is not, of course, without its dangers and no one involved in Christian ministry should be innocent of where these dangers lie.

Moreover, while those in secular counselling might not approve of touch as part of a relationship, for the Christian, touch is an important expression of love, especially where it is combined with prayer. Indeed I cannot imagine how, in a face to face encounter, prayer for another person can be offered without touch being involved. But while it can be an important symbol of love and intimacy in a spiritual context, in the wrong setting touch can so easily become a means of exploitation and abuse. Christian ministers need to be aware of these dangers if they are to allow themselves to be part of the culture of spiritual intimacy that Christian healing points towards. Power and abuse represent as great a temptation for the Christian as for any of the other people called to healing in the other cultures described in this book.

The prayer support for Christian ministry is in practice provided by a group of individuals who, in trust, are made part of the healing enterprise. Enough information can be shared with this group to make informed prayer possible, although obviously matters of great delicacy need not be communicated. I have found the work of such a prayer group of great value over the past ten years even when, as has happened, direct involvement of the kind I have described above with the sick has become less prominent in my ministry. The focus of the prayer group can then move more easily to be an intercession group for the parish, bringing the concerns of all the members into the prayer forum. Such a prayer support group is also vital for a healing service; without that kind of backing, healing services can so easily become over-formal and lacking in power and expectation. Sadly this scenario is, in fact, all too often the case. The reason is simply that the service reflects not the prayer of the people of God but the concerns of individual clergy or lay members who think, for whatever reason, that healing services are desirable .

In the healing relationship, a Christian will seek through love to create space for another person—space for them to express the deepest things in their heart, and space into which God's healing power can come. Whether the sick person is counselled by one or two people, there will be a quality or reality of love in the relationship which will probably not be paralleled elsewhere in their experience. It will be demanding on both sides as reality is explored, the reality of God's will and love for our lives and the reality of facing up to ourselves in our weakness and failure. T.S. Eliot declared that 'humankind cannot bear very much reality'. The Christian healing ministry is one that leads to reality, a simultaneously painful, transforming and healing encounter with the love of God.

Conclusion

The Christian healing ministry is both given and received within a setting or a culture which is uniquely its own. It takes as its norm the ministry of Jesus who mediated the kingdom power of God to the people of his time, a mediation which touched them with love, forgiveness and healing. The simplicity of his command to us to continue to 'preach the kingdom and heal the sick' is in practice compromised by many factors, both theological and practical. Few churches can hear this aspect of the church's mission, so it becomes conveniently shelved as too radical and challenging. But, here and there within the church, Christians do attempt to put into practice the command to heal the sick in proclaiming God's kingdom. From that activity, lives are changed and bodies sometimes healed. But the transformations and the healings that take place will always be somewhat muted. Because they take place within the setting of a particular culture, attempts to examine them in the light of another culture will probably be unsuccessful. Thus the power of God to heal rarely possesses a compelling quality to convince those who look at it from the outside. Jesus himself was not able to convince those who stood apart from his invitation to enter God's kingdom. Both the Christian faith and the healing that is at the heart of it remains a sign of a God who is involved with the world, close and gracious to those who belong to him.

CHAPTER 12

Conclusion

This journey through the contrasting cultures of healing in our society is complete. We have visited places on the map that perhaps we did not know existed. But in looking at all of these places together within the compass of a single book we can see certain patterns emerging.

In the first place we can acknowledge how the human body is a far more mysterious entity than any single model or system of thought in our society can understand. If we were to take even a little of the wisdom from each of these systems of thought in our society we would see we have something more intricate and amazing than the old philosophies have ever been able to show us.

If we do accept that each of the cultures has something to offer in helping us understand healing of the body and mind, we come to a second claim. And that is each and every philosophy of healing is incomplete if it cannot listen to what the other models of thought are saying. There is much evidence that there exist very few such bridges within our society.

The group of doctors who consider themselves practitioners of holistic medicine do appear to have created some important bridges between alternative thought and medicine. But even here I am not aware of any writing that shows that this group has shown any real understanding of Christian styles of healing. Christians themselves have not proved to be good bridge builders with other cultures. Many will pay lip-service to the culture of medicine while being resolutely condemnatory towards all other healing cultures. The paths of understanding between cultures will no doubt be slow to appear but perhaps this book will contribute a little if it can help you, the reader, to appreciate the wide interconnecting patterns of healing that exist now and will continue to exist in the future.

Christian healing

A final comment on the place of Christian healing amid the other cultures needs to be made. Although attempting to understand and communicate a range of healing styles that exist in society, this book begins and ends with a Christian contribution. Why is this? After all, attitudes on healing both within and beyond church boundaries have not been given a totally clean bill of health, and the frailties of the institutional church are well known.

The point is, the church follows a master who not only healed and told us to heal, he also exhibited in himself a model of 'wholeness' or healthiness that continues to inspire us.

In Christian healing there is an extra element in the answer to the question, 'What is health?' The conventional answer grapples with ideas of physical and emotional well-being; but for the Christian, the answer centres on an awareness of Jesus. To be whole in body, mind and spirit is to be like Jesus. It means imitating a constant rootedness in God and his availability and love for our fellow human beings. It means following him in using power only for the empowerment of others.

But following the wholeness of Jesus goes even further. It recognizes that the path of suffering may be also a path we are called to follow, and that suffering itself may be our means of finding wholeness and healing. To be a Christian involved in healing may take us to the very heart of pain, but we know that that place too has been blessed and hallowed by Jesus; there, too, God can give us his love, wholeness and salvation.

NOTES

1.   A discussion of the connection between medical practitioners and the pharmaceutical companies is contained in B. Inglis, *The Diseases of Civilization*, pp272–99. A recent article claims to have proved that hospital doctors are influenced by promotional spending by the companies.
M.-M. Chren *et al.*, 'Physicians' behaviour and their interactions with drug companies. A controlled study of physicians who requested additions to a hospital drug formulary.' *Journal of the American Medical Association* (1994) 271, pp684–89.

2.   H.K. Beecher, 'The powerful placebo', *Journal of the American Medical Association* 159 (1955), pp1602–6, cited in R. Ornstein & D. Sobel, *The Healing Brain*, Macmillan, 1989.

3.   S. Wolf, 'Effects of suggestion and conditioning on the action of chemical agents on human subjects: The Pharmacology of Placebos, *Journal of Clinical Investigation* 29 (1950), pp100–109, cited in *The Healing Brain*.

4 . H. Benson and D.P. McCallie, 'Angina pectoris and the placebo effect', *New England Journal of Medicine* 300 (1979), pp1424–29, cited in *The Healing Brain*.

5   R.W. Bartrop *et al.*, 'Depressed lymphocyte function after bereavement', *The Lancet* 1 (1977), pp834–39, cited in *The Healing Brain*.

6.   M.G. Marmot & S. L. Syme, 'Acculturation and coronary heart disease in Japanese-Americans', *American Journal of Epidemiology* 104 (1976), pp225–44, cited in *The Healing Brain*.

7.   H. Morowitz, 'Hiding in the Hammond Report', *Hospital Practice* (August 1975), pp35–39, cited in *The Healing Brain*.

8.   B.B. Arnetz *et al.*, 'An experimental study of social isolation of elderly people: Psycho-endocrine and metabolic effects', *Psychosomatic Medicine* 45 (1983), pp395–406, cited in *The Healing Brain*.

9.   See B. Inglis, *Trance, A Natural History of Altered States of Mind*, Grafton Books, 1989, p65.

10. A.H.C. Sinclair-Gieben & D. Chalmers, 'Evaluation of treatment of warts by hypnosis', *The Lancet* 3 October 1959, pp480–82, cited in *Hynosis for the Seriously Curious*, Kenneth S. Bowers, W.W. Norton and Co., 1976.

11. Y. Ikemi & S. Nakagawa, 'A psychosomatic study of contagious dermatitis', *Kyushu Journal of Medical Science* 13 (1962), pp335–50, cited in *The Healing Brain*.

12. L. G. Darlington & J. Mansfield, 'Food Allergy and Rheumatoid Disease', *Annals of the Rheumatoid Diseases* 42 (1983), 218. An account of this trial is found in *The Complete Guide to Food Allergy and Intolerance*, pp91–92.

13. J. Brostoff & L. Gamlin, *The Complete Guide to Food Allergy and Intolerance*, Bloomsbury, (2nd ed), 1992, p94.

14. J. Egger *et al.*, 'Is Migraine Food Allergy? A Double-Blind Controlled Trial of Oligoantigenic Diet Treatment', *The Lancet* **11** (1983), pp865–69, cited in *The Complete Guide to Food Allergy and Intolerance*.

15. Bang H.O. *et al.*, 'The Composition of Food consumed by Greenland Eskimos', *Acta Med. Scand.* **200** (1976), pp69–73 cited in D. Rudin *et al.*, *The Omega-3 Phenomenon*, Sidgwick & Jackson, 1988.

16 N. Hawkes, 'The Vast Potential of Fatty Acids', *The Times*, June 1994.

17 See J. Carper, *Food—Your Miracle Medicine*, Simon & Schuster, 1993, p27. The trial was carried out in the Tagore Medical College in India.

18 This trial is referred to in C. Wildwood, *The Aromatherapy and Massage Book*, Thorsons, 1994, p21. The researchers mentioned are Steve Toller and George Dodd.

19 See B. Inglis & R. West, *The Alternative Health Guide*, Mermaid Books, 1983, pp129–30. The researcher responsible is R. Melzack of McGill University, Montreal.

20 See B.Inglis & R. West, *Alternative Health Guide*, p130. They cite some research of the World Health Organization published in *World Health*.

21 This quote is ascribed to one Hiroshi Motoyama, the inventor of a machine which purports to read the meridians through electrodes. Quoted in *Alternative Health Guide*.

22 S. Parsons, *The Challenge of Christian Healing*, SPCK, 1986.

23 See D. Krieger, *Accepting your Power to Heal: The Personal Practice of Therapeutic Touch*, Bear & Co., 1993. Krieger is unusual in that she accepts testing and scientific scrutiny of all that she does. Her work is thus respected by a wide number of people who have seen the effect of her techniques which is of measurable efficacy. See T. Harpur, *The Uncommon Touch*, Hodder & Stoughton, 1993 for a Christian journalist's evaluation of her work.

24 A good up-to-date list of books on this topic is found in D. Cohn-Sherbok & C. Lewis, *Beyond Death: Theological and Philosophical Reflections on Life after Death*. MacMillan 1995, pp207–208.

25 See my account in *The Challenge of Christian Healing*, pp40–41. Also F. MacNutt, *The Power to Heal*, pp51–52.

FURTHER READING AND BIBLIOGRAPHY

The books listed below may be found useful for those who wish to follow up further the themes of each chapter. Those mentioned below will in most cases contain further bibliographies which will take the interested reader deeper into the themes introduced in each of the chapters. Experts on the various fields touched on in this book will no doubt miss other still more important works that are not mentioned. To them I can only say that the present work was written away from specialized libraries and the volumes available to the writer were those present in his own library.

Chapter 1

Calder, R., *The Life Savers*, Pan, 1961.
Coleman, V., *The Health Scandal, Your Health in Crisis*, Sidgwick & Jackson, 1988.
Currer, C. & Stacey, M. (eds), *Concepts of Health, Illness and Disease, A Comparative Perspective*, Berg, 1986.
Gordon, R., *The Alarming History of Medicine*, Mandarin, 1993.
Guggenbühl-Craig, A., *Power in the Helping Professions*, Spring Publications, 1971.
Inglis, B., *The Diseases of Civilisation*, Hodder & Stoughton, 1981.
Margerson, D., *Medicine Today*, Penguin, 1961.
McKeown, T., *The Role of Medicine*, Blackwell, 1979.
Medawar, C., *The Wrong Kind of Medicine?* Consumers' Association, 1984.
Melville, A. & Johnson, C. *Cured to Death, The Effects of Prescription Drugs*, New English Library, 1983.

Chapter 2

Bowers, K.S., *Hypnosis for the Seriously Curious*, W.W. Norton, 1976.
Chopra D., *Quantum Healing, Exploring the Frontiers of Mind/Body Medicine*, Bantam Books, 1988.
Collegan, M. J. & others (ed.), *Mass Psychogenic Illness: a Social Psychological Analysis*, Lawrence Erlbaum, 1982.
Cousins, N., *Anatomy of an Illness*, Bantam, 1987.
Coxhead, N., *Mindpower*, Penguin, 1979.
Friedman, H.S., *The Self-Healing Personality*, Penguin, 1991.
Marcuse, F.L., *Hypnosis Fact and Fiction*, Penguin, 1959.
Ornstein, R., and Sobel, D., *The Healing Brain*, Macmillan, 1988.
Sargant, W., *Battle for the Mind*, Pan, 1957.
Temple, R., *Open to Suggestion: the Uses and Abuses of Hypnosis*, Aquarian, 1989.
Torrer, E.F., *The Mind Game*, Jason Aronson Inc., 1986.
Watts, G., *Pleasing the Patient*, Faber & Faber, 1992

Chapter 3

Breggin, P., *Toxic Psychiatry*, Fontana, 1993.
Brown, D., & Pedder J., *Introduction to Psychotherapy*, Routledge, 1991.
Clare, A., *Psychiatry in Dissent*, Tavistock, 1976.

Dryden, W. & Feltham, C. (eds) *Psychotherapy and its Discontents*, Open University Press, 1992.

Eysenck, H., *Decline and Fall of the Freudian Empire*, Penguin, 1986.

Frank, J.D. & Frank, J.B., *Persuasion & Healing, A Comparative Study of Psychotherapy*, John Hopkins, 1991.

Hillman, J., & Ventura, M., *We've Had a Hundred Years of Psychiatry and the World's Getting Worse*, HarperSanFrancisco, 1992.

Kovel, J., *A Complete Guide to Therapy*, Penguin, 1978.

Masson, J., *Against Therapy*, Harper Collins, 1990.

Rogers, C., *On Becoming a Person*, Constable, 1967.

Chapter 4

Brostoff, J., & Gamlin, L., *The Complete Guide to Food Allergy and Intolerance*, Bloomsbury, 1992.

Carper, J., *Food—Your Miracle Medicine*, Simon & Schuster, 1994.

Chrystyn, J., *Life Force—the Secrets of High Energy and Optimal Health*, Smith Gryphon, 1994.

Hendler, S. S., *The Doctors' Vitamin and Mineral Encyclopaedia*, Arrow, 1991.

Mackarness, R., *Not All in the Mind*, Pan, 1976.

Paterson, B., *The Allergy Connection*, Thorsons, 1985.

Rudin, D. et al., *The Omega-3 Connection*, Sidgwick & Jackson, 1988.

Chapter 5

Benor, D.J., *Healing Research, Holistic Energy Medicine and Spirituality*, Helix, 1993.

Brennan, B.A., *Hands of Light, A Guide to Healing through the Human Energy Field*, Bantam Books, 1988.

Buckman, R. & Sabbagh, K., *Magic or Medicine? An Investigation into Healing*, Macmillan 1983.

Fulder, S., *The Tao of Medicine*, Healing Arts Press, 1990.

Fuller, R.C., *Alternative Medicine & American Religious Life*, Oxford University Press, 1989

Chapter 6

Gravett, P., *Making Sense of English in Alternative Medicine*, Chambers, 1993.

Inglis, B. & West, R., *The Alternative Health Guide*, Mermaid Books, 1983.

McIntyre, M., *Herbal Medicine for Everyone*, Arkana, 1990.

Salmon, J.W. (ed.) *Alternative Medicines, Popular and Policy Perspectives*, Tavistock Publications, 1984.

Trattler, R. *Better Health through Natural Healing*, Thorsons, 1993.

Vithoulkas, G., *The Science of Homeopathy*, Thorsons, 1981.

Wildwood, C., *The Aromatherapy and Massage Book*, Thorsons, 1994.

Chapter 7

Baker, R., *Binding the Devil, Exorcism Past and Present*, Sheldon Press, 1974.

Dearing, T., *Exit the Devil*, Logos Publishing, 1976.

Edwards, H., *Spirit Healing*, Herbert Jenkins, 1960.

Harpur, Tom., *The Uncommon Touch—An Investigation of Spiritual Healing*, McClelland & Stewart, 1994.

Harvey, D., *The Power to Heal*, Aquarian, 1983.
Peel, R., *Spiritual Healing in a Scientific Age*, Harper & Row, 1987.
Pilgrim, T., *Autobiography of a Spiritualist Healer*, Sphere, 1982.
Richards, J., *But Deliver Us from Evil, An Introduction to the Demonic Dimension in Pastoral Care*, Seabury, 1974.
Rose, L., *Faith Healing*, Penguin, 1971.
Rossman, M.L. *Healing Yourself*, Walker & Co., N.Y., 1987.
Sinason, V. (ed.), *Treating the Survivors of Satanist Abuse*, Routledge, 1994.
Tester, M.H., *The Healing Touch*, Barrie & Jenkins, 1970.

Chapter 8

Benson, H., *Beyond the Relaxation Response*, Fount, 1985.
Bohm, D., *Unfolding Meaning, A Weekend of Dialogue with David Bohm*, Ark, 1987.
Campbell E. and Brennan, J.H., *The Aquarian Guide to the New Age*, Aquarian, 1990.
Dossey L., *Healing Words, The Power of Prayer and the Practice of Medicine*, Harper Collins, 1993
Hampe, J.C., *To Die is Gain, The Experience of One's Own Death*, DLT, 1979.
Krieger, D., *Accepting your Power to Heal, The Personal Practices of Therapeutic Touch*, Bear & Co., 1993.
LeShan, L., *You Can Fight for Your Life, Emotional Factors in the Treatment of Cancer*, Thorsons, 1984.
McGuire, M. B., *Ritual Healing in Suburban America*, Rutgers University Press, 1988.
Miller, E., *A Crash Course on the New Age Movement*, Monarch, 1990.
Moss, R., *The Black Butterfly, An Invitation to Radical Aliveness*, Celestial Arts, 1987.
Osborn, L., *Angels of Light, The Challenge of the New Age*, Daybreak, 1992.
Perry, M., *Gods Within, A Critical Guide to the New Age*, SPCK, 1992.
Siegel, B. S., *Living, Loving and Healing*, Aquarian/Thorsons, 1993.
Siegel, B. S., *Peace, Love and Healing*, Rider, 1990.
Siegel, B. S., *Love, Medicine and Miracles*, Rider, 1986.
Simmons, J.L., *The Emerging New Age*, Bear & Co., 1990.
Smuts, J.C., *Holism and Evolution*, Macmillan, 1926.
Streiker, L.D., *New Age Comes to Main Street*, Abingdon Press, 1990.

Chapter 9

Arnold, D.M., *Dorothy Kerrin, Called by Christ to Heal*, Hodder & Stoughton 1965.
Brown, P., *The Cult of the Saints*, SCM, 1981.
Brown, P., *Society and the Holy in Late Antiquity*, Faber & Faber, 1982.
Cadbury H.J., *George Fox's Book of Miracles*, Cambridge, 1948.
Finucane, R. C., *Miracles and Pilgrims*, Dent, 1977
Frost, E., *Christian Healing*, Mowbray, 1940.
Frost, R.(E.), *Christ and Wholeness*, James Clarke, 1985.
Hendrickx, H., *The Miracle Stories of the Synoptic Gospels*, Geoffrey Chapman, 1987.
Hickson, J.M., *Heal the Sick*, Methuen, 1924.

Kelsey, M., *Healing & Christianity in Ancient Thought and Modern Times*, SCM, 1973.

Latourelle, R. *The Miracles of Jesus and the Theology of Miracles*, Paulist Press, 1988.

McCready, W.D., *Signs of Sanctity, Miracles in the Thought of Gregory the Great*, Pontifical Institute of Medieval Studies, Canada, 1989

Melinsky, M.A.H., *Healing Miracles*, Mowbrays, 1968.

Richardson, A. *The Miracle Stories of Jesus*, SCM, 1941.

Thomas, K., *Religion and the Decline of Magic*, Penguin, 1978.

Van Dam, R., *Saints and their Miracles in Late Antique Gaul*, Princeton, 1993.

Ward, B., *Miracles and the Medieval Mind*, Scolar Press, 1982.

West, D.J., *Eleven Lourdes Miracles*, Gerald Duckworth & Co., 1957.

Chapter 10

Davidson, I., *Here and Now, An Approach to Christian Healing through Gestalt*, DLT, 1991.

Gusmer, C.H., *The Ministry of Healing in the Church of England: An Ecumenical-Liturgical Study*, Alcuin, 1974.

Lewis, D. C., *Healing: Fiction, Fantasy or Fact?*, Hodder & Stoughton, 1989.

MacArthur, J.F., *The Charismatics, A Doctrinal Perspective*, Zondervan, 1978.

Martin, D. & Mullen P., *Strange Gifts, A Guide to Charismatic Renewal*, Blackwell, 1984.

Parsons, S., *The Challenge of Christian Healing*, SPCK, 1986.

Parsons, F., *Pool of Fresh Water*, Triangle, 1987.

Pattison, S., *Alive and Kicking—Towards a Practical Theology of Illness and Healing*, SCM, 1989.

Peddie, J.C., *The Forgotten Talent, God's Ministry of Healing*, Fontana, 1966.

Sanford, J. A., *Healing and Wholeness*, Paulist Press, 1977.

Sanford, A., *The Healing Light*, Arthur James, 1949.

Sanford, A., *Healing Gifts of the Spirit*, Arthur James, 1966.

Suurmond, J.-J., *Word and Spirit at Play, Towards a Charismatic Theology*, SCM, 1994.

Weatherhead, L., *Psychology, Religion and Healing*, Hodder & Stoughton, 1952.

Chapter 11

Bennett, R., *How to Pray for Inner Healing for Yourself and Others*, Kingsway, 1984.

East, R., *Heal the Sick*, Bethany Fellowship, 1977.

Glennon. J., *Your Healing is Within You*, Hodder & Stoughton, 1978.

Linn, D. & M. & Fabricant, S., *Praying with One Another for Healing*, Paulist Press, 1984.

MacNutt, F., *The Power to Heal*, Ave Maria Press, 1977.

MacNutt, F., *The Prayer that Heals, Praying for Healing in the Family*, Hodder & Stoughton, 1981.

Maddocks, M., *The Christian Healing Ministry*, SPCK, 1981.

Index